HOCUS POCUS LATELY

A Paranormal Memoir of a
Soon-To-Be Famous Anonymous
Artist as a Reluctant Healer
Or
Real Healing Lessons
From a Psychic Surgeon &
How You & I Can Do It Now

By
Valentino Zubiri

Books by Valentino Zubiri

Dollman The Musical
A Memoir of an Artist as a Dollmaker

Wonder
A Memoir of Relative Importance of a
Soon-To-Be Famous Anonymous Artist

Leadership Rubs: 1-Hour Mentors
A Memoir of an Artist as a Masseur

Hocus Pocus Lately
A Paranormal Memoir of a Soon-To-Be Famous
Anonymous Artist as a Reluctant Healer or
Real Healing Lessons From a Psychic Surgeon &
How You & I Can Do It Now

Healing Lessons from a Psychic Surgeon
6 chapters from Hocus Pocus Lately

**Valentino Zubiri: Nude Drawings &
Paintings from 1995-1996**

HOCUS POCUS LATELY

A Paranormal Memoir of a
Soon-To-Be Famous Anonymous
Artist as a Reluctant Healer
or
Real Healing Lessons
from a Psychic Surgeon &
How You & I Can Do It Now

BY
VALENTINO ZUBIRI

Hocus Pocus Lately, A Paranormal Memoir of a Soon-To-Be Famous Anonymous Artist as a Reluctant Healer or Real Healing Lessons From a Psychic Surgeon & How You & I Can Do It Now
First CreateSpace Edition

Copyright ©2014 by Valentino Zubiri
All rights reserved. No part of this publication may be reproduced, distributed or transmitted in any form or by any means including photocopying, recording, or other electronic or mechanical methods, without the prior written permission of the publisher except in the case of brief quotations embodied in critical reviews and certain other noncommercial uses permitted by copyright law. For permission requests please email valzubiri@gmail.com

Ordering information:
Individual orders: Amazon.com, most bookstores
Bulk quantity, trade bookstores & wholesalers: call first (312) 523-8052 or email valzubiri@gmail.com
Digital editions are available in various formats in most outlets online

Library of Congress Control Number 2014906355
ISBN-13: 978-1-4975-2094-3
ISBN-10: 1497520940

Printed in the United States of America

Cover & Book Design by Valentino Zubiri
Art Doll by Valentino Zubiri
valzubiri@gmail.com
vzubiridollman.blogspot.com
valentinozubiri.com
312-523-8052

"Hello Val, anak!"

"Hi Pa!"

Table of Contents

    Acknowledgments 1
1   Hocus Pocus Introduction 3
2   Fine Prints & Warning Labels 9
3   Psychic Surgeons & Fake Healers. 17
4   Dream About the Psychic Surgeon 23
5   Preschool & Mama. 29
6   Car Trouble. 37
7   Comic Books & Super Powers 39
8   The Apparitions of Cabra Islet 41
9   Liwanag. 47
10 The Spirit of the Glass 53
11 An Encounter at the Path 61
12 Intro-Version 67
13 College, Speedreading & the Girl. 73
14 An Incomplete Grade 77
15 Activism. 81
16 Star People. 85
17 The Prayer Continues 91
18 Superman & Other Thoughts. 93
19 The Hotel. 99
20 The Cook at a Restaurant 103
21 Aunt Li Getting Sick 109
22 Hocus Pocus Lately 115
23 Negatrons 119
24 I am an Artist & a Writer 125
25 Getting a Wish to Come True. 129
26 Marketing Study Points of View. 131
27 Papa Gets Sick. 133
28 Kansas City Danny. 141

29	Papa Gets Sick 2	145
30	Our Doomsday Generation	153
31	Repeating Numbers	159
32	Sinful Acts of Kindness	163
33	Envy	167
34	Lessons from a Psychic Surgeon 1	171
35	Lessons from a Psychic Surgeon 2	181
36	Lessons from a Psychic Surgeon 3	189
37	Lessons from a Psychic Surgeon 4	201
38	The Last Supper	219
39	Alien Abduction	227
40	Shadows & The Dream	233
41	Snakes in the Woods	241
42	The 1940s Psychic Healer	245
43	Vibrational Entities	249
44	Prayers	255
45	Neighbors	263
46	Jacks-of-All-Trade	277
47	Providence	295
48	Caring	301
49	Counting Our Blessings	311
50	Apocalypse & Armageddon	315
51	Convenience & Last Resort	325
52	Riddles	333
53	Words	337
54	How to Become a Psychic Surgeon	339
	Let's Connect Online	345

Acknowledgments

Papa, this is for you! Thank you!

This is also for Mama.

I also want to thank my siblings for being very supportive.

I also want to thank my friends Robert Siegel, George Mohovich and Jaime Almonte who have been very supportive.

I'm using my art dolls on the covers of three books which I am simultaneously releasing: **Wonder,** *A Memoir of Relative Importance of a Soon-To-Be Famous Anonymous Artist;* **Leadership Rubs: 1-Hour Mentors,** *A Memoir of an Artist as a Masseur;* and **Hocus Pocus Lately,** *A Paranormal Memoir of a Soon-To-Be Famous Anonymous Artist as a Reluctant Healer or Real Healing Lessons From a Psychic Surgeon & How You & I Can Do It Now.*

Chapter 1

Hocus Pocus Introduction

The late '80s to the early '90s. I decided to pursue art as a career in the late '80s. This was decades ago, and because I had also always wanted to become a writer, I came to the decision years later, in the early '90s, that I will write memoirs from the perspective of an artist.

The '80s. I was in college in the '80s, pursuing a BS Biology degree.

The '70s. Earlier, in grade school and high school, from the '70s and later, my dad, my brother and I read books about the more practical paranormal stuff, like dowsing using pendulums, developing ESP and pyramid power.

Today. It seems to me that, nowadays, more people entertain the strange. I had been planning to write about my paranormal experiences, but through the years, I could not seem to justify it, nor figure out how to approach writing about the more supernatural chapters of my life. Then in 2013, my dad got sick.

I had always been into the unexplained even as early as the '70s, and these past several years, I had also been listening to some paranormal radio shows, and I know that the weird is a popular subject and is part of pop culture.

I have come to understand that the audience is open to conjectures, because scientific information and study on the strange can be limited at best.

Because of this, I also believe that we writers should be very responsible and careful with what we tell such a receptive and welcoming audience. It is not so much as burning bridges for crying wolf. It is more because it can be easy to mislead the flock.

My challenge was that my most interesting strange encounter in my life was having spent time with a real Filipino psychic surgeon, a psychic healer, who allowed me to observe him for three and a half months and who actually taught me how he was able to do it. Unfortunately, this was also what threw me off.

I finished college with a BS Biology degree. I was one subject away from graduation when I met the psychic surgeon. It was difficult to make sense of something happening, right in front of me, that seemed impossible and contrary to years of lectures and laboratory work in the science pavilions.

What I saw was for a simple English term paper project, required for graduation, but this was the nail that stuck out. I did my best to graduate and then forget about psychic healing and psychic surgery altogether. It was too much for me.

Nowadays, I had gotten used to writing memoirs, and I came to realize that the best way I can convey my decades old "esoteric secrets" was through a memoir. With a memoir, I did not have to provide any logical nor scientific explanation nor proof. I can just write about my subjective thoughts because, at the end of the day, my subjective thoughts are all that I have.

I cannot provide anyone with a how-to on psychic surgery and psychic healing. In my opinion, it cannot work that way. All this, as you will discover, are mental and spiritual states that need to be maintained 24/7. This is not a job that can be turned on and off between 9 a.m. to 5 p.m.

I can only write a memoir and say, "Oh, by the way, I'm including the story about the psychic surgeon," and then say, "Oh, by the way, I *think*, I'm not really sure, but I may be a healer myself, and this is how I *believe* I did it."

This book is a collection of my weirder stories, still part of my Memoirs of an Artist Series. I'm a little thankful that some stories did not directly involve me. I don't think anyone would remain sane and coherent if all the stories I have here involved the same person.

Having become familiar, lately, with the shows and the listeners of the paranormal talk shows, I figured that if I wanted to write a book for such an audience, I should do my best to make it a one-shot, so this book is thicker than my other memoirs. There are a lot more stories here, and I actually retold a few important stories from the other books, within the context of leading into the more mysterious explanations.

I figured, readers who would be into this field of UFOs, crop circles, chupacabras, prophecy, ghosts, psychic power, and, psychic healing and psychic surgery, just like myself, would want this book, while readers who are into the arts and myself as an artist would continue to entertain and read all of my books. Hence, this has become a thicker, one-shot book.

This book will play "catch up." Some stories here, from the Philippines, will compare to the current goings on in other countries.

For example, we have all seen shows about UFOs in the U.S., Mexico, New Zealand and Australia. It's almost impossible that the Philippines would have nothing that is UFO-related. The country is located around where Australia and New Zealand are.

I graduated with a BS Biology degree, so obviously, I do understand scientific approaches. Topics like these in the book cannot easily have explanations ready. The best way I can approach this book was to make it into a memoir. I would have my valid reasons.

First, I'm used to writing memoirs. I set deadlines for myself to come up with four memoirs by this time in 2014. This book was part of my plan. I had to write a memoir before anything else, including a how-to, which would be challenging, considering that I cannot provide complete proof of anything mentioned here even if I wanted to.

Second, I can share my written stories without stopping to think if I was being objective and scientific enough about anything. I don't have plans to produce pictures nor graphs.

Third, a memoir would enable me to write about *all* of my thoughts about the events, because at the end of all this, without providing anything scientific, this is all I can really provide you in all honesty.

I have never invented a story in my other memoirs, and I would not want to do it in this book. I understand that we who are into the metaphysical and unearthly are more open to theories than the average person, and as such, I know I should be careful with what I want to share with you.

I graduated with a BS Biology degree in 1986. Obviously, my education was based on science. It was a pre-medical course. I had been entertaining becoming a writer then, but the prospects were bleak because I was in the Philippines and I wanted to get published in the U.S.

I was already into the paranormal then, so I took the chance to write about Filipino psychic surgery for a simple English term paper—my last writing hurrah before I graduated.

As you can see, it took me 28 years to even begin to write about this again. If I wanted to fool you, I would have done it sooner. Maybe I want to fool you now. I'm kidding.

It turned my world upside down. It was *that* strange and powerful! Why would I write something that would make other people question reality to the point of self-defeat, unproductivity and insanity? Well, I didn't really go crazy here.

To reword, I used to be uncomfortable with the subject, so why would I write something that would make others uncomfortable as well? "Used to." Not anymore. I can now share with you what I know in a more stable way.

What made me write this, as you will discover is that I believe I got signals from somewhere unknown that told me it was time to write about all this. A conjecture, but valid enough for me.

I also believe that with a huge audience, you, the reader, especially if you're into the paranormal, will not be as alone as I was in the past, thirty years, or twenty-eight years ago to be exact, when I was just so rattled by the experience, at the time of my graduation, when I was supposed to proceed to medicine and I decided not to, that I just simply decided not to mention it to anyone, including my own parents and siblings, and friends. I shut it out and forgot about it.

I got a grade of 'A' on my term paper, as expected. Throughout these years, I hoped that it was shelved and forgotten. Now I'm writing about the experience, together with other experiences in a more informal way.

This is why I will begin my next few chapters with warnings. I want you to be prepared.

What might be different and more positive with your experience, however, is that it is now the 21st century, and we have all become a little more open to possibilities that do not need full explanations.

What is also different this time, is that I am sharing this book with a huge audience. It will not be like my old term paper that was solitary, it left me with questions and a change in my paradigm without the support of other people.

Despite this book, which I believe is the only book that details how a genuine Filipino psychic surgeon was able to train himself to do what he was able to do, I will continue to claim that all this is conjecture, and that faith will remain faith, and will continue to have difficulty becoming fact.

Remember the time of Christ. He miraculously healed people. Two thousand years later, we never arrived at how he was able to heal, nor was it ever duplicated on a massive scale that by now western medicine should not have even evolved.

So expect something, but not everything, from **Hocus Pocus Lately**. It's a memoir of an artist as a reluctant healer. I obviously used the term "Hocus Pocus," because as I have said and will continue saying throughout the book, all this is difficult to prove, there are no clear destinations and pit stops, but it's a strange enough ride.

Chapter 2

Fine Prints & Warning Labels

I'm calling this early chapter, "Fine Prints & Warning Labels."

In contracts and medicine boxes, you see fine prints and warnings. Fine prints and warnings are there, but the powers that be don't seem to want you to see it.

When you meet a person for the first time, you are at a curious, but wary, stance. You want to move forward with the interaction, on the one hand, and on the other, you mind is looking for ways to relate to and judge that person. You are a little observant and critical. You are looking for meaning. That is what I mean about "fine print."

"Warning labels" are when I mention my own doubts.

Going back to the example of meeting someone for the first time. If you noticed that person's suit is a little off, maybe it's old or a little too short or too long, if you begin thinking that the person is probably financially hard up, but is doing his best, then that would be fine print. At the same time, you become cautious, you start to think that he might ask you for a favor, maybe ask you for some money, or maybe something else. That would fall into the category of a warning label.

༄

Here is a major combination of fine print and warning label.

The psychic surgeon was a Christian. What's the fine print? If you ask yourself, "How come I'm Christian, and I can't do psychic surgery or psychic healing?" That would be fine print for you.

If you tell yourself, "Uh-oh, he's going to convert me right now, this early," then you just gave yourself a warning label.

At this point, you go back to your fine print mode and ask yourself, "I wonder what lessons I might be able to use for my own, despite the fact that I'm Buddhist, or into new age or Muslim?"

So fine prints here happen when you continue on and proceed and analyze the situation. When you stop and see something that is off to you, then those would be warning labels.

☙

Why do I sound cryptic? It is because we are dealing with the abstract here. We are doing something "psychic," but based on my experience, and based on the teachings of the psychic surgeon, this is a psychic or mental state. This is not a 9 to 5 job. This is a challenging 24/7 mental state. The only way it can manifest is if your whole existence is shifted.

My memoir is about me. I cannot tell you which exact part led me to where I am at, and I am also telling you that what I can do probably might not compare to what you or someone else will be able to do.

I probably did a few things which I believe can dissipate psychic power. But it's part of my life and this is a memoir.

What you might find that I did right will become your fine print. What you might find that I did wrong will become your warning label.

☙

Beyond fine prints and warning labels, are what I call "Riddles."

Riddles will be your own questions to yourself. After you read this book, you will continue to have questions. Like what I say, this is not a how-to book. At the same time, don't expect a how-to book on how to live your life 24/7 just so you can manifest psychic healing. It would be like asking for a CliffsNotes version of the Bible that you can read and follow with assurances that you will still enter the gates of heaven.

The other supernatural stories are here, because they are part of my own supernatural experiences. While this book has a lot of chapters about healing, this is still my paranormal memoir.

☙

So now, I'll tell you the fine print about the other paranormal stories.

The major fine print is that these are part of my set of experiences that have led me to my set of beliefs. As I encountered each one, I was led to believe that they do happen and they do exist. You will get a feel of my psychology, of how one thing led to another. As you read them, being that you know I'm not lying, nor did I invent these stories, then maybe they can be your springboard if you want to become a healer.

I'm not asking you to paraphrase what you read in this book, I'm asking you to become more sensitive to your own surroundings, your own thoughts and your own life, if you want to see if you can develop the gift of healing as taught by the psychic surgeon. This book is my story and yours will be different. Look at this book as a springboard.

If you have no plans to become a psychic healer, then just enjoy the book.

☙

I've been going to Catholic mass quite regularly lately, and I will mention this many times later, but for now, as an example of fine print exercise, let me show another example.

I went to a weekday mass. There were only about 20 people in the huge church.

There was a Gospel reading where Jesus encountered a blind man who asked to be able to see. Jesus healed the sick, and as the man was walking away, Jesus told him to walk home, and not towards the village. The priest gave his sermon afterwards.

As the Gospel was read, my own interpretation was that Jesus told the man to go another way, because Jesus did not want the village to come rushing to him to be healed of their afflictions. This Gospel was read just a few days ago.

I was obviously with the mindset of writing and finishing this book. Being that teaching the readers how to heal was the concept in my head, I cannot wait to tell this story, because it appeared that even Jesus was reluctant to announce his healing ability. It was not his time to become known. That once-blind man would had represented him in the way he did not want to be perceived as of yet.

The same thing was happening with me. Even after having experienced some parts of this book over 30 years ago, I still hesitate about writing all this. You should hesitate as well. I'm not a healer as much as I'm a storyteller, just telling you these things. I probably should stop writing about healing, but I had made a decision to do so, and I could still be wrong about all this.

As I listened to the Gospel, I put myself in the shoes of Jesus, and then in the shoes of the blind man. Jesus seemed to be unsure if the once-blind man should let people know Jesus can work miracles. The man had proof of healing. He probably would had gone to the village to tell every person there. These were my thoughts as the Gospel was read.

Then the priest talked.

He concentrated on Jesus telling the once-blind man, "Take a different route! Don't go to the village." He pretty much said, you might find yourself in a bind, and if things aren't working well for you as you do what you think is right for your life, then take a different route!

See how different his interpretation was?

As I was in my own mindset of "fine print," my mind churned again, as I began to interpret what he had to say! I wondered, if the priest knew I was writing this book, would he tell me to stop? My current route was to write this book.

So here is an example of looking for fine print in life as related to God and/or the Law of Attraction, whichever is better for you.

I was being sensitive, entertaining the thought of receiving my own cryptic messages from the Cosmos or God.

Even as I try to be specific with this example, you might also realize that by being in that mindset, I was expanding my psyche, however you might want to define that.

Did Jesus just tell me, through this priest, to stop writing it? As you can see, this was part of my everyday life, there was nothing paranormal or supernatural about that day, it was my mindset that was working here.

What was also funny, the reason I was relating this to myself, was the fact that I had become a familiar face to the priests. I started going to daily Catholic mass on a daily basis around October 2013. As I wrote this second chapter, it was late February 2014. (I started to write some chapters of this book in May 2013.)

Confession at this church was face to face. Time came when I had sat with all the three priests assigned to the church. Confession this way was pretty much an informal chat session. I had shown pictures of my doll art on my cellphone to them. This winter had been brutal, with more days under freezing temperature than the past years. As a result, there had been some days when only 15 people showed up for daily mass! It was very easy to see a familiar face, like mine, and indirectly advise me through the sermons. Or maybe this was just my interpretation.

☙

There was the other priest whose sermon another day was to make sure to start getting things done and goals accomplished. Once again, there was only a handful of us, and he had just heard my confession a few days before, during which I showed him the progress of my contemporary art dolls, my target financial reward and my joke that I would be able to pay for the repair of the church's leaky roof, if only I succeed soon!

☙

So this is me reading my own fine prints, or reading between the lines.

I'm just encouraging you to do this early on. What I'm saying is, as you read my book, become more and more sensitive. As you go through life, notice, more and more, the invisible. Notice my fine prints, and notice your own fine prints.

If you want to learn to become a psychic surgeon, or psychic healer, then you will need to read my memoir to analyze what I may have done right and what I may have done wrong. So there's your fine print related to this book. Some stories about what happened to me, which I wrote as a memoir, reflected the teachings of the psychic surgeon.

Then you look up, you stand up, and you begin becoming aware of your own fine prints in life; things that seem invisible, but are there.

☙

Warning labels are more grounded. They would be more basic.

I studied principles of hypnosis and neuro-linguistic programming informally for more than two years. At home, I watched videos, listened to audio lessons and read books. My goal was to improve as a writer. I improved but I'm also still learning more.

(By the way, I'm not a full-fledged hypnotist nor an NLP practitioner. I'm just knowledgable.)

What is related here is that hypnosis and neuro-linguistic programming—the use of choice words for life change—have a common tip: Stories are told to make people remember the lessons better than had a list of tips and pointers been given. This obviously serves my purpose. A memoir is a group of related stories.

What I call warning labels are those stories that seemed to have a lesson of being careful. If I debunked my own experiences, there would be a warning label somewhere, whether implied or stated.

Some warning labels would be obvious. For example, I have a chapter where this man went to poop in the forest, at night, and he got bitten by a snake and died. There's a warning label.

Don't go to the forest looking for UFOs or bigfoot, with your head in the clouds, thinking you would become the most famous, well-celebrated, most talked about person on the planet, without reminding yourself that there are more immediate dangers lurking in the vicinity. Venomous snakes, spiders, scorpions, poison ivy, a serial killer, mosquitoes.

Here's another relevant warning label related to the story. I was letting you know how difficult going to some parts of the Philippines can be. I did not state this outright.

The man came home to the island with the snakes to show his parents his diploma. The fine print was honoring his parents. He needed to show his parents his accomplishment, but he failed to be careful.

Another fine print: My dad told me this story. Through the years he had discouraged me from returning to the island, where he was born, to become a farmer or something else.

It could also be prophetic, coming from my dad, that if I came home to him, I would die. Maybe it was his way of accepting that he and I were okay communicating over the phone, separated by the Pacific Ocean, halfway across the world from each other.

☙

My worry for you is that this book might change your paradigm. It is a memoir of an artist as a healer. As you go through my life and thoughts, you will also come to learn how psychic surgery in the Philippines is done.

I had always known that I had to write this book. I want you to take things first with a grain of salt, like warning labels. As you read more, and you get more ready, then you can begin to look for more and more fine prints.

Chapter 3

Psychic Surgeons & Fake Healers

Before you read on, I want to define some similar sounding terms I pretty much stick to. I'm defining them for the purposes of you understanding this book. These are my own definitions as I proceed to write this book, not an expert's. Well, I could be the expert, but let's not worry about that right now.

It is important to mention these terms early on in the book. I'm also telling you that I had been aware of these terms through the years from other sources, but I'm not quoting them.

By the way, when I mention something from the Bible, I will not tell you exactly where it came from. I'm not trying to convert you. I'm writing a memoir and in this book, my narrative can be fanatical enough. I will never ask you to open the Bible.

☙

Here are four terms: *faith healing, fake healing, psychic healing and psychic surgery.*

Faith healing is when someone talks about God, and then as part of his or her ministry, will ask God for healing for an individual, a small group, or the entire congregation. We see this on television.

Fake healing is a comedic play of words, used because the word "fake" sounds like "faith." So if someone deliberately claims to be able to heal, but knows in his or her mind that he or she is only deceitfully claiming it, then that would be fake healing. I do not think that this definition should include the belief of the patient, because the placebo effect can still take over. We are referring to the "healer's" dishonesty for this one.

Psychic healing is when someone talks about healing through

the mind and unseen forces without involving God. If God or religion is mentioned, it would only be in passing. Laying on of hands without the mention of God would be psychic healing.

Psychic surgery is when someone claims to have some sort of psychic power or ability and is able to open skin and astonishingly close it back up in a strange and obviously, still unexplainable, way. The definition of the term can vary with people. Here is where psychic surgery as defined by myself will differ from psychic surgery as defined by others.

☙

There is a Brazilian man who is known as "John of God," He is very popular because through the years, he has been the only person in Brazil who is supposedly a psychic surgeon. His popularity has reached the United States and other countries, and so, internationally, the popular world definition of psychic surgery seems to be based on his practices.

The thing about John of God, is that he uses sharp tools to make incisions. On YouTube, I saw him stick a forcep up into the nose of a person and twist it about! Needless to say, I was shocked. His practices vary from those of a Filipino psychic surgeon.

He might be a psychic surgeon, but the definition, when referring to him would include elements which Filipinos don't have. He supposedly allows other entities to enter and use his body to perform actual surgery on the patients.

I am from the Philippines. Filipino psychic surgery usually refers to the process of skin opening up without the use of anything sharp at all. A wound is produced, the psychic surgeon is then able to probe inside the wound, and once the session is over, the wound closes up without sutures. I have actually seen the psychic surgeon's hand go inside a patient's abdominal cavity, all the way to his wrist! I saw beforehand that the skin had no openings. I also saw afterwards that the skin closed back and the wound had disappeared. The psychic surgeon did not use anything sharp; he just waved his hand.

Wikipedia states that "Psychic Surgery" is, a "pseudoscientific procedure typically involving the pretense of creating an incision using only the bare hands, the removal of pathological matter, and finally the spontaneous healing of the incision."

Know too that the following is the immediate next paragraph in the Wikipedia entry:

"It has been denounced by the US Federal Trade Commission as a "total hoax," and the American Cancer Society maintains that psychic surgery may cause needless death by keeping the ill away from life-saving medical care. Medical professionals and skeptics classify it as sleight of hand and any positive results as a placebo effect. It first appeared in the Spiritualist communities of the Philippines and Brazil in the middle of the 20th century, and it has taken different paths in those two countries."

Please read the entire entry by going online. Please read other websites about psychic surgery as well.

If you are convinced that it is a hoax, believe that you are right. You would actually be better off for it, and so you can stop reading.

I agree with some parts of the entry. The placebo effect could be happening. I will explain more throughout the book.

༺༻

As a writer, whoever put that on Wikipedia already had presuppositions.

"Presupposition" is a term in hypnosis and neuro-linguistic programming. It means that as you say something new, you hint at something else in the sentence or sentences that are already accepted as true.

For example if I say, "As soon as you use our product, you'll finally be happy with your oven." A presupposition here is the assumption that the customer was never happy with the oven in the past. There is also the presupposition that the product being sold has not yet been used by the customer and that the beneficial result has not yet been observed. Because of these presuppositions, the speaker subconsciously invalidated the customer's past good experience with the oven, placing the customer to question if he or she was even ever happy with the oven in the past.

Going back to the Wikipedia entry. Whoever put in the words "pseudoscientific" and "pretense" in the definition already had a negative attitude towards psychic surgery.

"Total hoax," versus just using "hoax" obviously no longer allows for anything else. "Denounce" sounds like, "We are taking a stand, we have already passed judgment, with or without proof, you should be on our side, or face ridicule."

The mention of the Federal Trade Commission and the American Cancer Society seems to add credence and power to the harsh words used. They seem to discourage people from finding out for themselves.

I do believe that psychic surgery has a lot of flaws *and* I saw it genuinely performed. I'm being cautious here. I used the word "believe," because I'm not basing anything on any proof. I also stop at the fact that it was performed, but I'm not following it up with testimonials, claims and proofs from the "patients" that they really got cured.

Writing is a play of words. The attitude of the writer is reflected.

〜

Here is something that can add to the confusion. I have a hunch that Christ 2000 years ago did psychic healing. I believe that psychic healing as Christ did it, was so strong that there was no more need for psychic surgery. If this were the case, then we are focusing on something that is high up but at a level that is just below what Christ was able to do.

If we start playing with words and circumstances again, in the eyes of a religious person who had witnessed real psychic surgery, that Wikipedia entry would sound blasphemous. It will seem as if there is no more room for Jesus Christ to be back in our current, modern, westernized society.

I hate to add to the confusion some more, and to flip-flop between sides, but I would still side with western medicine if we continue to get headlines of people, especially children, who died because the parents believed that their strong faith would save their loved ones' lives without the need for doctors and hospitals.

∽

As I discuss psychic surgery, psychic healing or faith healing in this book, be reminded that there are no proofs provided. I have a bachelors degree in Biology, and I myself will prefer to undergo chemotherapy and radiation therapy if I were diagnosed with cancer.

Modern medicine exists because it has been proven to increase chances of success in dealing with illnesses.

However, at the same time, I might want some faith healing for myself as well. Maybe even psychic healing and psychic surgery. It would not hurt to have someone lay his or her hands on me if I were sick. I would probably trust a psychic surgeon to do his or her "hocus pocus," but only after I had seen him or her do it on someone else.

∽

I will keep reminding you that the main purpose of my memoirs are for my long-term goal, of becoming known as an artist. I would rather tell small, stupid stories that define me; I would rather write honest stories. I would not say I saw a flying saucer, if I only *thought* I saw a flying saucer.

∽

Back to my definitions. A Filipino psychic surgeon, is obviously already defined as a psychic healer, because his purpose of doing psychic surgery is to heal. A psychic healer, if he or she cannot do psychic surgery, cannot be a psychic surgeon. Usually, before a psychic healer or psychic surgeon administers to his patients, he talks about his Christian beliefs and his Christian God, and if he tells the listeners that what he can do came from God, then the healing has a hint of faith in it, and it becomes faith healing.

The reason why the term "faith surgery" is not used, is that by the time psychic surgery occurs, there is physical manifestation, clearly seen, and the power of the mind, without the need for faith to be part of the definition, is acknowledged. The manifestation went past invisible belief into what the eyes can witness.

In this book, I will freely, interchangeably use faith healing, psychic healing and psychic surgery. These terms can be used on the psychic surgeon I met, because he claimed to have obtained his power from his Christian beliefs.

Here is our main presupposition for this book: I did meet a psychic surgeon who was not a fake one. For almost 4 months, every Sunday, I was next to him when he did what he claimed to be able to do. You will have to believe this in order to go forward with this book.

Definitions. Don't think I did not think this through. I did. I want to share with you as much thoughts, conjectures, knowledge, mysticism, religion and mystery as I can. I want you to learn and at the same time get entertained. I try to be objective while being subjective. Once in a while I debunked my own experiences. I myself sometimes expressed disbelief in what I wrote about.

Chapter 4

Dream About the Psychic Surgeon

One night, a dream. The man in front of me was a Filipino whose name I had chosen to forget. When I dreamt this one, I knew it was a dream, I knew I was asleep, and it came as a surprise that I knew I was dreaming.

"Do you remember everything I told you?" he asked me.

"I'm sorry, it's been so many years, and I am still afraid. It scares me to even think about it," I said.

"What do you remember?" he asked.

"Oh, stuff," I said.

"Do you still remember me?" he asked.

The dream stopped there. This dream happened three times in 2001.

I guess if I were to continue with a memoir, I would have no choice but to dig in a little deeper into my past. Back in 2001, I was starting to entertain my first memoir about my days as a masseur.

I went to college and acquired a Bachelor of Science degree in Biology. That was a scientific study. On my third year, I became interested in Economics and Business Administration. I thought about shifting. I did not want to become a doctor anymore.

However, because most of my courses were for Biology, it would had taken me six years or more to shift and finally get an undergraduate degree in another field.

Thanks to Mama, I realized that I was better off finishing Biology, then going for a Masters in Economics or Business Administration.

Well, my four-year Biology degree took me five years to complete, and my transcript was laden with red marks which meant that I didn't pass some courses the first time I took them. I especially had to take some science courses three times. Failed-failed-passed.

On my fourth year, I had an incomplete course, English 2. I missed a requirement for the grade, a term paper. I had to come up with a term paper over the next year to make the grade and finally graduate.

In my search for alternative directions in life other than medicine, I made a decision to shock myself, by making a term paper on psychic surgeons.

Psychic surgeons are psychic healers in the Philippines. They claim to open up skin with just their bare hands, take out tumors or blood clots from their patients, and close up the wound with just the power of their will. No scars were supposedly left.

In researching about them, I had to venture out of the school, and since I led a sheltered life of school, home, classmates and friends, I had to shock myself into introducing myself to and meeting people outside of school.

So I did my initial research through books, and then I had to search for a psychic surgeon to interview. I acquired several phone numbers, of male and female psychic surgeons. Finally, it turned out that there was a weekly "healing service" conducted near my home, just less than an hour away.

Since I didn't drive, I used the jeepney, the city's public transportation.

I saw a crowd gathered in a home, a lot of people spilling into the sidewalk. That must be the house, I thought. I walked past a few people, and into the compound.

The center of the gathering was in a garage that was without any cars. In it, I saw benches and many people, most of whom appeared to come from below average incomes—poor, by the way they dressed. There was some sort of desperation in the air. A plea for help and healing from people who could not afford a doctor, or who were probably told that their conditions were incurable or costly.

There were three six-foot tables, in front, looking much like altars, I thought, but a person laid on each table. Overlooking each table was a healer. Assisting each healer were at least two other persons.

From my observation, there seemed to be at least four healers taking turns on the three tables.

I saw a man with a friendly air about him, who seemed to manage things near the entrance. I approached him as he saw me and he approached me as well. I started to ask questions.

"Why do the healers take turns?" I asked.

"They get weak and need to rest," he answered.

"Is there any way I can talk to a healer afterwards? I'm researching for school."

"Yes, you can do that. Which school are you from?" he asked.

"University of the Philippines. It's just for my English term paper."

"I noticed you didn't seem to belong here. So you're from a good school," he commented. I knew what he meant. I understandably dressed a little better than the rest, because I went there as an interviewer. I also did not look sick.

"Oh, thanks," I said, referring to his comment about my school. "Do you think I can talk to one of them?"

"Yeah, but maybe not today. Two of the four doing the service today are supposed to go out of town to another place, and they also get weak doing this. They might not be willing to engage themselves in an interview."

"What about asking for an appointment for later?" I asked.

"That will be a problem. Some are going out of town for a few days. However, I will be available tomorrow." He said, smiling, like he thought his answer was funny.

"What do you mean? Are you telling me you're also a healer? How come you're not over there?" I asked, smiling back.

He smiled back again, and said, "Yes, I'm also a healer. I'm having a service tomorrow."

"Here?"

"No," he said. "I just help out here every Saturday. Mine is at my house on Sundays."

"Are you a healer or a psychic surgeon?" I asked.

"Psychic surgeons are healers," he said.

"Yes, but can you do psychic surgery?" I insisted.

"Yes, I can," he answered.

"So—" this was it, I told myself. "Can I interview you?" I asked him.

"You can tomorrow," he said, "but not here, because it's not my territory. I don't want to insult my colleagues here."

"Okay. What time and what's your address?"

The man began to write on the notebook I handed him.

"Try to come an hour earlier so I could talk to you before the service," he said.

"Are you going to tell me how you do it?" I asked, as he wrote his name, phone number, address and service schedule.

"Sure, why not. I'll tell you what you want to know," he said. "5 p.m.—service." Then he wrote "4 p.m.," and encircled it.

"Okay, I'll see you tomorrow then. Is it okay if I observed these people today for the meantime?" I asked.

"Yes, just go towards the front," he said. "They wouldn't mind."

"Thanks."

I went to the front and observed. I didn't want to ask any questions of doubt yet. Observing, I noticed that the healers' hands were clenched, as if they were concealing something, like oh, maybe bloody chicken fat, pretending to get something from their patients.

But as I glanced at one of the healers, a man whose hand was over an old lady's exposed belly, I noticed his hand come up from the belly, and I saw a hole on the belly. Then the hand came down on the gaping hole, then came back up again, and the wound wasn't there anymore!

I waited for another instance like that again, but I never got a second chance. I was already a little shocked. An hour and a half later, I felt things were getting a little redundant. Healers and patients got their turns on the tables. I decided to go home.

I said goodbye to the man I was going to see the next day, and went out through the gate.

I sat by the driver's side on the jeepney. Jeepneys have a mirror that ran the length of the front behind the driver's rear-view mirror, part of the vehicle's customary design. I looked at my reflection and saw myself flushed. I had the look of uncertainty and self-consciousness. My heart was racing.

It could be that I was in an unknown territory. I had ventured out of my school. I saw real psychic surgery happen. I had stayed in front of the crowd, self-conscious, as usual.

But the most shattering of all, I felt as if all my four years of scientific study in college, plus this fifth year of overstaying, had just come crashing down.

Chapter 5

Preschool & Mama

My second and youngest sister, Amelia, the fourth sibling in my family, was born about 6 years after my first sister, Dinna. For a while there were three of us. My brother Jing was the oldest, then I followed, then my first sister, Dinna. The three of us, Jing, myself and Dinna were approximately a year apart from each other.

Dinna at age 3 stayed at home together with our housemaid, the hired help, while my brother and I went to this certain school, which only had prep and kindergarten. My brother was placed on the prep level, while I was placed on the kindergarten level. I never compared books with my brother, but my first box of crayons only had a single row of 8 colors. His was 16, in a box with 2 rows. My brother was 5 years old; I was 4.

Mama went to school with us. My class did not have walls. It overlooked the playground. I saw Mama sitting with the other moms and nannies, talking to them, smiling. They sat in rows of benches facing the playground. Sometimes she crocheted. The other mothers and nannies crocheted as well. Whenever I craned my neck to look for her, if I didn't see her anywhere, I cried my eyes out.

My brother's class was a little farther, and more hidden, with walls, far from the seats where mom was. He never cried for Mama. He was stronger than I was.

By lunchtime, classes were over, and the three of us went home. We took a taxi, but once in a while, we walked.

Mama crocheted. She made doilies and displayed them at home. Decades later, I learned to knit. She never learned to knit, I did. I never learned to crochet, at least not yet. We discussed this frustration once in a while now. I had this idea to learn some sort of a trade every year. More than 10 years ago, it was December, and I had not yet learned anything. Knitting occurred to me because it was winter and I thought I should learn to knit a sweater. The knitting store nearby sat me down for 3 hours.

What Mama and I never discussed was that she introduced me to the paranormal, in a very indirect way.

⁂

I remember Mama taking my brother and I to a new place, where this lady administered a test for my brother. I remember the lady looking at me. I remember myself innocently acting shy and obedient, avoiding her stare.

She looked at me then talked to Mama.

I heard Mama saying I was supposed to go back to the preschool, where I would be placed in the Prep class. My brother was to go to this new place, a bigger school, and so, therefore, yes, we would be separated.

The lady said it did not make sense for Mama to be going back and forth between two schools.

Mama said the idea was for me to be a year lower than my brother, to save money. I was going to use my brother's hand-me-down books, maybe even his uniform. The first year of us being separated was a worthwhile sacrifice for her.

I was told this plan earlier, and I thought it was a smart decision by my parents. My brother and I shared most of our clothes. The cost of the books were the issue. My parents told us we were poor. The lady, however, said that although my age was still a year too young, since I was already there, I might as well give the entrance exam a try.

Mama looked at me, and told me I was going to take the test my brother just took.

I took the test. I completed a few mazes, matched sets, encircled images of fruits and geometric shapes which did not belong with the rest, etc.

Then we walked home. From that walk that probably took 45 minutes, until all those succeeding hours when we were home, until the time Papa arrived from work, I remember that the topic was about the new school, and that I took the test prematurely. I might not pass anyway.

I think that was in March or April. School was out. All this was in the Philippines, when school started in June and ended in March, just before Holy Week.

By May, Mama told my brother and I that we both made it in.

By June, on the first day, Mama took us to the big school. I was placed in Section A and my brother was placed in Section B. The prep level in that school had 6 classes, Section A to Section F.

On that first day of school, I learned that the students in all the grade levels, from prep to seventh grade, and all the way to high school, were classified according to their intelligence, based on grades. Mama explained it to my brother and I.

For about a month and a half before this Day 1 in the new school, I was in limbo. I did not know where I was going to be placed. I had finally learned not to cry in the kindergarten, and I was looking forward to using the swing in that playground. I finally got the courage to swing as high as I could muster the energy to do so. The slide was a different story. I stopped going near it. One of my classmates thought it was fun to get up on the platform at the top of the slide, and pee, while the parents, nannies and teachers laughed at the disgusting sight. I never got on the slide after that incident.

So that period, summer vacation, I was thinking about my preschool a lot. I had become familiarized with some of the names and faces of my classmates and I was wondering who would be back, but now I might be displaced and be placed in the new school, on the same level as my older brother, whom, although we were just a year apart, I respected, because he looked bigger, older and smarter than me.

We followed a generational system in the Philippines, used among siblings. An older brother would have a prefix, *Kuya,* ("coo-YAH") before his name; an older sister would be called *Ate* ("ah-TEH"). So we younger siblings call our oldest brother, Jing, "Kuya Jing." Kuya Jing calls me "Val," but my two younger sisters call me "Kuya Val." My younger sister, Dinna, is Dinna to Kuya Jing and I, but is "Ate Dinna" to our youngest sibling, Amelia, whom we three simply call Amel. Jing is a nickname. His real, full name is Fernando. My full name is Valentino. Dinna is just Dinna.

Mama, on Day 1 in that huge school, took us to class. She took my brother to his class. Section B. Then she took me to my class. Section A. She asked me if I want for her to stay with me. I told her no. I was in the Prep level, the level my brother was in last year. Kuya Jing never needed to see Mama like I did. I told her to go home. I was going to be okay. She laughed. I remember her smile and her eyes that day as she looked at me to ask that question.

My class was air-conditioned. The doors were closed. The teacher introduced herself, as she wrote her name on the blackboard. We had a piano on the side, which she played. I thought the piano must be why our classroom was air-conditioned with the door closed. It was cozy. I noticed that the other classrooms, including where my brother was, were not air-conditioned. I did not feel special. I thought about my brother. He was older, he should be here in my classroom. I thought, had I not been admitted to that school yet, had the original idea been followed, he would have been sitting where I was.

Lunchtime. School was over. The entire school seemed quiet. We were told to keep quiet because the higher levels still had class till the afternoon. Mama picked us up and we walked home.

I asked why I was Section A and Kuya Jing was placed in Section B. I was being considerate.

Mama answered, "They probably made a mistake with your names and got confused with your sections."

During that school year, I seemed to have blanked out. I

wanted my brother to be smarter than I was. My mind somehow drifted, I daydreamed a lot. Sometimes, in reading class, I saw letters but not words.

A year later, Dinna started going to school. Mama spent time with her. Same thing, but this time, Mama took her to a different school and sat with the other new moms and nannies. This was a new preschool a few more blocks away from my previous preschool, and the familiar teachers from my preschool were stolen by that new one.

On the next level, Grade 1, my brother was placed in Section A. I was placed in Section B. It felt good that I successfully found my place again in the family. I vindicated myself, even though I didn't have a word for it then. While in Grade 1, I saw my brother get high grades. I studied harder. My next goal was to become classmates with him from Grade 2 and onwards in Section A.

෴

Back to Mama. Through the years, it was either Mama or the current housemaid who was in school, either to bring our lunches or pick us up. Sometimes Mama was there during lunchtime, to bring our lunch, and she then waited with other mothers and nannies until class was over.

One time, Mama went home with a small plastic bag of fried, obviously cooked, but greasy, brown-colored grasshoppers. She showed them to me, and she started eating them, asking me if I wanted to try some. I shuddered and made a face.

"Why would I eat grasshoppers?" I asked, wincing.

"They're not grasshoppers, they're locusts," she corrected.

"Where did you get those?" I asked.

"One of the moms promised to give me some. She's from a different province and they eat these where she's from," she explained.

Mama hung out with the other moms and nannies, where they were allowed to sit—at the cafeteria, which we Filipinos called the "canteen," or on the benches under shady trees, on one side of the huge quadrangle, that the J-shaped, 4-story building encircled, or the benches encircling that one huge tree, still in the quadrangle, but nearer the canteen. The quadrangle was for everyone, from Prep to Grade 1 to Grade 7. The younger levels ran around the quadrangle playing Cops and Robbers or Tag. I observed that as the Grade level got higher, the students got tamer. The fourth floor, which had Grade 5 to Grade 7 was the most orderly.

High school, which was something I did not have to worry for years, was the next building across a side street.

༜

Papa brought his work home with him. He always had piles of papers, which he said were "income taxes." He had a mimeograph machine. There were no copiers then. This was in the '70s. We sometimes helped him with or watched him work the mimeograph machine. He typed the forms first, on some sort of mimeographing paper using a manual typewriter. He was fast, forceful, and noisy, when he typed. He also typed just as fast and forcefully when he had to type on regular bond paper, or when he needed to use carbon paper for duplicates and triplicates. I guess my brother and I got used to Papa's typing sound, the speed in which he typed, to become fast typists ourselves. Papa was high tech. He churned out forms from the mimeograph. Xerox was not around yet.

༜

Back to Mama. We were still kids, but we remember days when Mama cried in the bedroom, blew her nose, cried some more. We asked why, and she always said she and Papa had a fight.

Our family lived in a big house in Manila, owned by Papa's parents. We never moved out of there. It appeared even bigger because there were small residences that my grandparents rented out cheaply to about twenty impoverished households. We called it *looban* ("loh-OH-bahn"), the "inner" residence, which were on the northern and eastern walls of the compound. Although each residence had their own bathroom, the water supply came from a single, central faucet. Water wasn't scarce in the city, but there was a meter. My grandparents had to make sure water wasn't wasted. By the time I was in Grade 2, all the residents, except for one family, tailors I will mention in a later chapter, and their three kids, were made to leave. It was 1972, when Martial Law was put in place. My grandparents thought new laws might be put in place where the residents would become difficult to oust.

Our huge main house was halved, my grandparents lived on one side, and my family lived on the other side.

Through the years, Mama had her in-laws to contend with. No matter how hard she tried to be okay with them, they didn't like her much. There was a time when a housemaid of my grandparents told them, that she overheard Mama, and my older first cousin, Ate Yoly, our housemaid at the time, plotting to poison my grandparents! Of course, that was a lie, but that did not stop my grandparents from giving Mama the silent treatment for at least a couple of years. My grandparents' envious, evil servant, was a younger sister of their other servant. The older girl told them the accusation was a lie and that her sister was a bad seed. We suspected the girl wanted to be on my grandparents' good side.

My grandparents always hired people who come from their island, Lubang Island. With Martial Law came the hearsay that land in the Philippines was going to be taken and redistributed amongst the poor. Everyone wanted to be on my grandparents' good side. They wanted the best land that they can get for free. That girl eventually left them, and the last thing we heard about her, by the time I was in college, was that she was prostituting near Clark Air Base, the American army base in the province of Pampanga, about 2 hours from Manila.

☙

Back to Mama. Around Grade 5, I noticed that Mama started bringing home stapled, mimeographed copies—text which she had been reading.

On certain days, she told us she was going somewhere and will be back soon. Then she came home with some more mimeographed copies.

I finally asked what those copies were about. There were religious statements, starting with "My beloved children," or some other similar phrase.

Mama said they were transcripts from this lady who supposedly had been seeing the Blessed Virgin Mary. On certain days, this lady opened her home to a few people. She and the visitors prayed together, then she went into a trance to talk to the Virgin Mary. Mama initially got the transcripts from one of the moms who hung out at the school. Then Mama started going to the lady's home herself.

After a few months, I finally asked Mama if I can go with her.

I went a couple of times. The house was nice. People knelt and prayed the rosary, the lady was at the front and center of the group nearest an altar with religious statues. Everyone faced the altar as they prayed. Then the lady went into a trance, turned and faced the rest. Next to her was a man, with pen and paper, writing down what she said, as supposedly dictated to her by the Virgin Mary.

I think after a while, the novelty wore off for Mama. She stopped going.

Mama had kids she needed to raise. She was a housewife. Although through the years she and Papa got into home-based moneymakers on the side, like baking cakes and muffins and even raising a hundred hens in cages for their eggs, built where the demolished looban slum homes were, she probably felt trapped. She lived with her in-laws who disliked her, had fights with her husband, and there were years when she had no hired help, no housemaids nor houseboys. During those times, she had to hand wash, hang dry and iron our clothes, clean our side of the house including the bathroom, and cook our food—everyday. She probably thought she was never appreciated. She was depressed and looking for connection with a higher power.

Chapter 6

Car Trouble

I too was looking to connect with God.

As I mentioned in my other memoirs, I had my conflicts stemming from my feelings of inferiority to my brother, not to mention the fact that I noticed my dad did play favorites a good number of times through the years.

My once-in-a-while thoughtless actions included crossing the street in Grade 1.

We were walking home, Mama, Kuya Jing and I, just a block away from school. I ran, crossing the street ahead of my companions. I lost my balance and stumbled onto the street. A car almost hit me. The bumper stopped right in front of my face.

The driver immediately got out of the car, picked me up, a lady in the back opened her door, I was put in the car, followed by my mom and my brother.

I was taken to the emergency room of the same hospital where my mom had given birth to the three of us. Amel was to be given birth there as well in about a year and a half. A doctor examined me. I was not hurt.

To cut the story short, as I have extrapolated on this incident more lengthily in my other memoirs, I remember my mom telling me and my brother to keep this a secret from Papa. I told her I was not hurt, why wouldn't we tell Papa.

She said Papa would *kill* her if he learned about this one. I distinctly remember her telling me that Papa would "kill her," she said that in our Filipino language. I knew it was a manner of expression, not to be taken literally. Still, I faulted myself for one of the first secrets I had to keep from Papa at a young age.

By second grade, they hired a houseboy, not a girl. I was molested by him for about 4 months. I would not blame him, though. I also blamed myself. Another secret to bear. It made me all the more introverted for the years to come—the rest of the elementary school, high school and college. At that age, I thought that I was the world's only victim of such a thing.

I would not talk about this any more than this paragraph above. I talked about this in other books, maybe I will mention it again in future books. Needless to say, I embarked on a search to correct my existence that spanned more than a decade. Like my mom, I had my own vacuum inside me.

Chapter 7

Comic Books & Super Powers

Papa liked taking us to the bookstore.

I got Papa to buy me my first American comic book during the summer break between Grades 2 and 3. It was a local reprint of *DC's Adventure Comics* which at that time featured Supergirl. Like any other young nerd, I wished I could fly. I thought superpowers would take me away from the unhappy childhood I was in.

After the usual collection of Hardy Boys and Nancy Drew detective books, as we got older, we got into the paranormal. In school, from Grade 4 to Grade 6, my classmates had paperbacks and hardbounds about witchcraft and ghosts. UFOs became a popular subject for my classmates by Grade 6.

By Grade 6, my dad, Kuya Jing and I went to the bookstore and got paperbacks on pyramid power, dowsing and other paranormal subjects, which to Papa seemed more practical.

The maids during those years, my mom's and my grandparents', used to read the local Filipino comic books. Mama discouraged us from reading those, but I loved the horror stories. The local comic books were weeklies, not monthlies, so the addiction to the stories were satisfied on a weekly basis.

∽

There was a regular ad in the local horror comic. There was a local store in Manila that sold talismans! I was intrigued. I think I was in the 4th grade when I insisted for Mama to take me to that store! The ad was a mail order ad. They listed the talismans available, what they could do, the prices. Cash, checks and money orders were accepted for mail orders, and there was an address! Superpowers! I had to go to that store!

I begged and pleaded with Mama for months to take me to the store. I cannot ask Papa, he would not approve. She kept telling me those items were fakes, the ad was fraudulent, and the address was too far. Then she finally relented. She took me there, to appease me.

We took at least two jeepney rides. The jeepney is a form of public transportation in the Philippines, which usually looks like an American Wartime Jeep in front, but the back is elongated. The front can squeeze in 2 passengers, while in the back passengers sat on the left and right sides on long seats that faced each other.

Nowadays, you can Google "jeepney" to see how they look. They are very colorful and well-decorated.

Back to the story.

Mama was not lying. I just had to check out the talismans for myself, before spending money. I too had my doubts.

The ride was long. Although it was still in Manila, the location was too far away from home. We also had to walk on an unpaved, muddy road. The house was a poor man's house. The locale was poor.

We were allowed in by this tall, middle-aged man with a pot belly. He asked us to wait in the living room. He disappeared through a doorway that was covered with a bad-looking fabric that served as a curtain. He came back with a few of the so-called talismans. Some were as large as a small-sized cookie, all made of metal. If my memory serves me right, the charms seemed like they were made of pewter. The designs had crosses, but nothing seemed Catholic.

I lost interest, because I thought I remember seeing that one of the talismans on the comic book ad was for money and prosperity. I thought another one was for becoming attractive and irresistible, and this guy looked creepy. We thanked the man for showing us his products, and went away. On the way home, I thanked Mama for taking me there. My curiosity was satiated.

Chapter 8

The Apparitions of Cabra Islet

Around 1976, my family was at some social function, in a restaurant in Quezon City. Someone stood up, my family knew him from my school. He spoke about God. Then he mentioned this island in the Philippines where he saw miracles in the sky and the apparition of the Blessed Virgin Mary several times. He mentioned that there was a yearly pilgrimage to that island, or islet, every December. It was under the auspices of President Marcos, the same person who gave us Martial Law in 1972, at the request of his very old mother, who was by then in her eighties.

When we went home from the function that night, Papa talked about the island. He said he too had been there on the island in the late '60s. We three siblings were too young to go, he said, but he and other relatives did go there and witnessed strange events. Us kids were left in Manila.

So this interesting subject was opened up after about 8 years of silence. Once in a while we asked Papa and the cousins of his whom he went with, when they visited us at home, to describe what they saw. It was a lively topic, they all lit up describing the paranormal.

They said, a group of girls saw a glowing lady, floating several feet from the ground, several times. She eventually identified herself as the Blessed Virgin Mary, mother of Jesus Christ. It happened on Cabra Islet. This started in December 1966. I was born in 1965.

Cabra is Spanish for "goat." It was said that only goats can be raised there, because the normal farm animal, the carabao, the popular Filipino word for the water buffalo, would be useless there. The island was big enough to have it's own public school, but not big enough to have enough farmland for a carabao to be raised in. Goats eat grass, including weeds.

By 1968 or 1969, like Fatima, a special day was announced, when the apparitions would be spectacular. My dad and his cousins went. I think my grandpa went as well.

They said the people prayed. The visionaries were there by the special tree where the Blessed Virgin occasionally appeared. Then the sun and the sky behaved in a strange manner, they saw bursts of color in the sky. The blue sky changed to a variety of hues.

Then a huge white man, who looked like Santa Claus, with white hair, white beard, and blue eyes appeared, and he was so tall, the trees did not reach his knee. He was smiling, looking at the crowd. Then he started to approach them as he set the trees to the sides with his hands.

The crowd panicked. Papa thought there was this giant who might step on the crowd; there was no place to run because the crowd was huge. Then in an instant, the giant disappeared.

Other people, according to Papa and his cousins, either saw the same thing, or something else, or nothing at all.

Cabra Islet was easy access for Papa and his relatives, because they grew up on Lubang Island. Lubang Island is a tiny island that is part of Occidental Mindoro.

Cabra Islet is part of the municipality located on Lubang Island. Papa and his relatives had homes and farmland on Lubang Island.

By 1976 a week after that social function we were in, I bought a book on the apparitions of Cabra Islet. The book was thick, with supposed signed testimonials by numerous witnesses through more than 5 years.

In December 1976 of that year, we went with the pilgrimage. Papa, Mama, Kuya Jing and myself. We boarded a grey-colored Navy boat, which left Manila in the evening. It was a free trip as it was sponsored by the government.

We pretty much camped out on the deck. We had sweaters,

jackets and blankets. We saw the man who talked at the function. We had our bags of food for the trip. We slept through the night, using additional blankets for pillows.

We were awakened by the rising sun. As I surveyed my surroundings, I saw other people waking up as well.

There was a lady who had a wavy kris, a decorative, shiny, wavy sword which she held in front of her as she concentrated, with eyes closed. She was with another lady who looked sick. She touched the lady with the kris, as if she was knighting her, on the head and the shoulders. Then she prayed again.

We figured she must be a faith healer.

Then Cabra Islet was seen on the horizon. As we neared, everyone prayed the rosary. The ship anchored about two miles from the shore. Small Filipino-styled motorized *bancas,* we called them motorboats, approached the ship to take us pilgrims to the island. It took hours for everyone to patiently empty out of the boat and get on the island.

I looked at my watch. It was 11 a.m. My family was still on the ship. We were one of the last ones to get off. Everyone continued to pray the rosary in unison as we waited for our turn on the small motorboats.

What was striking, and I'm sure that there is a scientific explanation to what transpired, was that as the sun rose, everyone prayed looking straight at the sun. The sky was clear, all blue with not a cloud in sight. Throughout those hours of prayer, we were looking straight at the sun, and it was not blinding us. There seemed to be a gray filter in front of it.

Still, our eyes probably furthered the trick, because it seemed as if the gray filter was a gradual of an inch smaller than the sun. It seemed to move, or dance in a circular manner. That must have been because as we stared at that one object, our eyes probably involuntarily moved a little.

Once again we camped overnight, this time on the island, near the apparition hill. We walked around the island during the daytime, praying where the group prayed. I saw the legendary cross that I read about in the book I bought.

A tall cross made out of aluminum square tube was erected at the apparition site, at a clearing near the tree. According to the book I read, this supposedly metal cross swayed, on occasion, from side to side, to its left and to its right, as if the vertical bar were not made of hardened metal. Like rubber, the vertical bar bent, so that the horizontal ends touched the ground. This cross was tall, and made taller by a base made of cement. It did not sway when we were there.

In the afternoon, we walked around the islet avoiding where it was steep. It definitely was a small island. It did seem that goats were the ideal animals to raise there.

In the early evening we visited some homes, whose residents Papa knew. I think some of them were our distant relatives. At one time while we were relaxing in one of the homes, there was a commotion. Some people rushed to the hill. We were too tired to bother. When we rejoined the crowd later to camp out for the night, we learned that some people claimed to have seen a ball of light descending from the sky, heading to the apparition hill.

According to the book I had read, many different witnesses did see balls of light on different occasions. From Lubang Island, for example, a group camped out and viewed the island through a pair of binoculars. They saw lights, as if a procession was being held, moving around the island. However, one of them saw Christ carrying a cross at one point, which the others did not see.

Another group of witnesses, through binoculars, claimed to have seen the Virgin Mary gliding where there were trees. They saw the trees bowing to the Virgin as she floated.

☙

The book I read, with plenty of testimonials, also included at least one person seeing a sash floating in the air, where the apparition tree was. The sash was tied to the waist of an invisible person. It seemed to come in and out of focus and turn invisible as it moved to the left and to the right, as if the invisible wearer seemed to walk about.

To me, the way it was described, it behaved as if supernatural performers were preparing for a show, but forgot to turn off a switch, as the audience, the human beings, began showing up.

I kept that thought to myself. No one else in the family read that book anyway.

☙

On the next day of that pilgrimage to Cabra Islet, the pilgrims, the adventurer (my brother), the superhero (myself), Mama, Papa, and the rest of the pilgrims from Manila once again got ferried to return to the naval ship by the few motorboats that belonged to the locals and their enterprising neighbors from nearby Lubang Island. This was an annual event, an opportunity to make some money. The ferrying was a slow process that started in the afternoon at around 3 p.m. We were, once again one of the last to board it. It was past 8 p.m. For a while we worried that the ship might leave us behind.

The ship left Cabra Islet. The island's silhouette got smaller. All of us looked at the islet and up at the star-filled, December night sky. We were hoping for one last strange event, which never took place. The tiny lights generated by the candles, gas lamps and Coleman gas lanterns in the homes that dotted some parts of the island got tinier and dimmer.

The next morning, we were back in Manila and the pilgrimage was over. It was December. My brother and I missed some school days for this great, strange, although mostly uneventful experience, except for the nonglare of the sun. The next event I was looking forward to was Christmas break.

Odd, but we never bothered to tell our classmates where we were. We never saw anything out of the ordinary. We thought any rising sun probably wasn't blinding to begin with.

On my freshman year in high school, I submitted a science experiment to my science teacher. Supposedly, milk didn't spoil but instead turned to yogurt when placed under a cardboard pyramid aligned to true north.

I can't remember how the topic changed when I talked to my science teacher as I submitted to her my project, but I eventually told her the story of us going to this place called Cabra Islet. I told her my family saw the nonblinding sun, but the book I owned told of other occurrences. The way I talked to her was animated as if I was in awe. Talking about it did not feel right, and so for many years I never talked about Cabra Islet again.

☙

The following year, we went to a party. We saw my dad's acquaintance again. We asked if he was going back to the island on the navy ship. My brother and I were eager to go back just because.

He said no. He said it seemed that other forces might be at work. It could be UFOs or other types of beings that could be misleading us.

I can't really agree nor disagree with this analysis.

At a young age, if I saw a tall aluminum cross that behaved like rubber, I probably would be a much different person right now.

It was probably for the best that we did not return to Cabra Islet.

Chapter 9

Liwanag

Sometimes, my grandparents, Papa's parents, hired our distant relatives from my grandpa's side to be their household help or housemaids. Gina and Liwanag, sisters, were two relatives we liked to have around, but they took turns being in Manila. Their brother Dodi, used to be one of our playmates when we spent our summer break on Lubang Island.

Gina had shoulder length black wavy hair. She looked more urbanized with her hair that looked permed, but some Filipinos have naturally wavy hair.

I had always thought Liwanag, which is a Filipino word meaning "bright" or "brightness," as having the likeness of a deity, a Filipino goddess, first because of her name, which was very Filipino, and second, because of her long, silky, straight hair that usually reached her waist.

Liwanag was older than Gina, probably the oldest sibling. She sometimes tired easily. She mentioned a few times that she had asthma.

They had another sister, Benida, who was also about my age, who grew up with their uncle and his wife, more distant relatives. I think Dodi followed Benida. They had a shy older brother, who never hung out with us.

We kids were usually on the island with our grandparents as soon as school was out in March, just in time for Holy Week or the week after.

The small town where our grandparents lived in was Tilik, which was the island's port town. It got busy on the days when the small ships from Manila arrived and left. Our house was just around the first big intersection from the small pier. We had no television, and electricity was intermittent, turned on only a few hours during the day. When the electricity came on, the old refrigerator hummed, and it ran just enough to produce an old, muggy smell that mixed with the island's fresh, salty air, flavored by the sea. The water did not cool down and we didn't care much for producing ice in the freezer.

We only had the radio as our connection to Manila. It was always on AM, which had the native language talk shows about Filipino matinee idols, and dramas, including horror at night, which the islanders and us listened to by the dim kerosene lamps.

We usually hung out with one or two kids our age. There was a beach front towards the west end near the town's small cemetery, that was shallow in the afternoon when it was low tide, littered with living corals and shiny seashells, mostly cowries, starfish and brittle stars. Dinna and I used to go there, through the gate of another distant relative, in the early afternoons, to check out the marine life. Collecting shells got old after a while.

On the island, around the time when my brother and I hung out with Dodi and another friend Bert, we sometimes saw kids clapping and tiny mists flew out of their hands and up into the air.

We learned the trick and I did it a few times, but we were warned not to do it too much, because the "mists" can get into our lungs.

Benida showed us how it's done. Kerosene, used for the gas lamps and bamboo torches, and chewing gum. Once the gum started tasting bland and the sugar is gone, wet your palms with kerosene, and mix the gum in with the kerosene until the gum starts spreading all over your palms. Start clapping. After a while the gum separates from itself into tiny particles that the wind will carry. Keep clapping until all of the gum is gone and up in the air, or until a neighbor shouts for you to stop.

The adults on the island did not like this activity. First, they said that the gum can get inhaled and get stuck inside the lungs, and second, the gum can stick to the houses. True enough, at a later time that summer break, I saw my gum start sticking to a wall and some trees. I stopped doing it, although it was fun and tempting to do.

I thought, if Benida enjoyed doing it as she demonstrated it to us, maybe Liwanag, when she was younger did it as well. Some probably got stuck to her lungs.

Years later, Gina was the hired help. One time, we watched a show on television. There was a man who talked about dwarves. These dwarves, according to the dwarf expert, were short, invisible beings, who liked to live in the provinces, but some lived in Manila.

They are not to be disturbed. Some people accidentally pee on strange mounds on the earth, or on the side of a seldom-used path. They get sick the next day, supposedly having been cursed by invisible spirits, some of whom can be these dwarves.

Gina started getting excited. She said those dwarves did exist, and she told her interesting story.

Some years ago, Gina said, Liwanag disappeared for many days from their home. They looked for her everywhere and weren't able to find her. They finally gave up, hoping she would return.

She did return, groggy and disoriented, as if she did not know where she was.

For a few days, she did not talk. When asked later on, she said it felt like she had only been gone a few hours. She was taken to a kingdom where the dwarves were.

These dwarves did not look human. They were short. They had tough gray skin and big, round, black eyes. They did not speak, but communicated using their minds. Liwanag was with them for a while, and then she was returned.

She was found wandering, wearing the same clothes when she disappeared days before. She was weak and incoherent for a while, unable or unwilling to talk about the experience. She finally talked about it days later.

They did believe her, Gina said, because they believed that

interaction with invisible, other worldly beings did happen. Where else could she have gone anyway. It was Lubang Island. Everyone knew everyone else. Liwanag would know if she were simply kidnapped by a neighbor. The town of Tilik had a few square kilometers of residential blocks.

And Gina added that something peculiar also happened a few days after they found her. They had a pet cat. Liwanag played with it once, basically playing with the cat on her lap and petting it, or teasing it. The usual things people do with cats. The next day, the cat was found dead.

Gina said it was not some type of a permanent curse that was with Liwanag. It seemed that Liwanag looked weak and drained of energy for a while. She eventually recuperated, but remained sickly on occasion. Whatever it was that affected her, it affected and killed the cat. Liwanag insisted to sleep away from them when she was found, and Gina said maybe that was for the best. They also thought she looked unpredictable anyway. They thought she was insane.

☙

As I grew up, Liwanag was the tallest amongst her siblings, and being the oldest, she was the first to mature. My sister and I liked to hang around her whenever she lived in our house in Manila as our grandparents' maid. She used to comb her long hair, and, from the base of her scalp, she pinched her hair a few strands at a time, tracing them all the way to the tip. I thought this practice of hers made her hair silkier.

There was a time when we kids started to scratch our heads. Mama said we had lice. I mentioned Liwanag's practice of pinching her hair. Mama said people did that if they had lice! Liwanag had lice and she gave them to us. I thought she was a goddess. I thought goddesses did that to keep their hair silky straight!

Mama told us to do our best not to hang out with her too much. I think Mama bought a fine tooth comb for her to use. As the maid, stuck in Manila, she had no relatives willing to search for lice on her head. Had she also been on the island it would have been easy to wet the hair with kerosene, while staying away from fire, when bathing. Kerosene kills lice.

I came to the United States around three decades ago. I'm an older man now. I learned that Liwanag finally had a really bad asthma attack and died.

☙

Now, having seen documentaries on aliens and UFOs, I think Liwanag may have been abducted by gray aliens. She was statuesque. If I was a gray alien, Liwanag, on nights of candles, kerosene lamps and torches, brighter Coleman gas lanterns and primitive-looking bamboo torches, being on a remote island, separated by the unending sea, amidst all that fresh air and the rustling of coconut fronds that danced with the breeze, she was a good candidate for impregnation with alien hybrids.

Those beings were bald and hairless anyway. They probably were unaware or did not care about her lice.

Nowadays, in my mind, she remains a goddess.

Chapter 10

The Spirit of the Glass

Around 1990, I got a Ouija board from a resale shop, in Chicago. I bought it together with some $10 used suits that fit me. Well, I eventually got an office job that did not really require those suits. The friend of a friend type of contact paid off.

I had just started hanging out again and making new friends then. While at my home with a few new friends, I took it out. Only one agreed to use it with me. With two fingers on the planchette, the planchette moved a few times. I was skeptical and amused. I thought the other guy moved it. There was no way to ascertain. We put it back in the box. I never used it again. I eventually threw it out.

I actually found this American version too small, without much space to move about. However, the gimmick of the American Ouija Board, that probably makes it sell well, is that the board *is* meant to be small, making the setting more intimate and snuggly for the teenage users. It has its purpose.

The Philippines is not without its version of a Ouija board.

☙

Papa did not just bring his work home. During the times when he worked in Manila, on weekends, he used to like to drive to his bosses, coworkers and work-related friends. He used to bring us kids with him. I guess he was playing office politics. Then again, he also brought us to Mama's relatives. Papa had really good p.r.

One time, he was assigned a higher position, but it was in Oriental Mindoro, the eastern side of the big island of Mindoro.

The main Mindoro Island is so huge that in the '50s, it was split into two provinces, Oriental Mindoro, the eastern half, and

Occidental Mindoro, the western half. Before his job assignment, the huge Mindoro island really did not have much impact on our family.

The patches of agricultural land and beachfront properties my grandparents owned were on the tiny Lubang Island, part of the province of Occidental Mindoro. Lubang was so much more backwards then. There was also a direct route from Manila to Lubang. To get to Lubang Island, we simply drove to Manila's North Harbor, Manila's pier for domestic ships, hopped on board one of those small-sized ships, slept overnight on cots, and directly reached Lubang Island. The island's pier is located in Tilik, a few houses from our grandparents.

A cot per passenger was important, because travellers used up the space underneath for all the luggage they can bring from Manila—suitcases, boxes, huge cans of cookies, woven baskets and there was never a trip that did not have a chicken clucking or a rooster crowing. Heading back to Manila, the luggage get an additional trove of huge baskets of mangoes and *sineguelas,* also called Spanish plums in other countries, and sacks of rice in summer and citrus fruits in December.

We kids used to race to the house, our bags carried by some of our grandparents' workers. There was really nothing prestigious to all this. We either needed to throw up or needed to use the bathroom.

By the way, the name Mindoro was coined by the Spanish colonizers, from *mina de oro,* or "mine of gold." Don't ask me where the gold is.

The big island of Mindoro, with the two provinces, Oriental Mindoro and Occidental Mindoro is more urban, with restaurants, stores, paved roads, cities, movie houses, water supply—less boring, although it still did not compare to Manila.

Papa left us in Manila to work in Calapan, the capital city of Oriental Mindoro, but he went back and forth between Calapan and Manila to be with us whenever he can. To get to Calapan, he had to take a 6-hour bus ride to Batangas Port, in Batangas, another province south of Manila, then hop on a 45-minute ferry boat ride to Calapan.

His boss came from the city where he was assigned to work, so before he was able to find an apartment, he stayed at his boss' old Spanish style house.

Papa had a cousin, *Tito* Aton ("Uncle ah-TAWN." His real name is Arthur.), who was younger than Papa. Tito Aton back then was not yet married. At some point in the future, he became Tito Nick's, or Uncle Nick's driver, but he eventually went to work in Saudi Arabia with his future wife, *Tita* Emma ("Aunt Emma"). Tito Nick was one of Papa's brothers.

Tito Aton pretty much hung out at our house in Manila. When Papa went to Oriental Mindoro, in the city of Calapan, he followed Papa.

Papa needed a companion to stay with him at his boss' big, empty house. No one else lived there. Papa needed to work to keep us afloat, that was obvious, but his sacrifice to leave us in Manila to make the moolah led him to live in a haunted house!

His boss' grandiose old-style villa that Papa said seemed to had been built during the Spanish era, probably around the 1800s, was not just old and unused when they got there. It did not just serve as a home for his boss' family, but it also served as a Japanese army headquarters during World War II.

Tortures and death were never far behind during the Japanese Occupation. Maybe some Japanese prisoners were tortured, held or died there.

One of Calapan's pride is a martyr who is awaiting sainthood, Wilhelm Finnemann, who was originally from Germany. He was appointed as a titular bishop for Calapan. He was arrested by the Japanese during World War II for refusing to turn some schools and convents into places for comfort women and brothels with underaged girls.

The Japanese arrested him under the pretense of jailing him in Manila, but they threw him out into the sea between Calapan and

Batangas.

Tito Aton told us that at night they heard noises inside the huge old house. It sounded as if people were moving about. He heard some items and chairs move. For the most part, he covered himself with his blanket, and only on occasion dared to try to see what was going on in the dark. Papa did the same. They both also saw things that not only moved, but floated in the air.

I guess Papa needed to accumulate enough money before he was able to move to a more normal apartment.

Tito Aton went back to Manila around the time when Papa moved to an apartment.

Mama went to see Papa and stayed with him for days, sometimes weeks, leaving us in Manila with our maid who managed our meals, clothes and school. Our grandparents were on the other side of the house anyway, with their own maids, so we were not really alone.

☙

Or maybe it was the boss' daughter who caused the hauntings.

Papa said the daughter liked to play "Spirit of the Glass," the Filipino version of the Ouija board. See, the manufacturers of the American version never got to the Philippines. They would not have succeeded, since the Philippines was predominantly Catholic and very religious. The outspoken religious would have prevented the Ouija board from getting marketed there.

☙

What Filipinos do is make their own homemade Ouija board.

They invert a regular drinking glass to use as a pointer. The letters and numbers are written on a large piece of cartolina, which is paper the size of a posterboard that is as thick as cardstock. This is why I thought the American version was too wimpy and small.

It turned out that even his boss' house in Manila had spirits. The daughter supposedly played Spirit of the Glass, probably with her friends, attracted spirits but, according to Papa, probably did not know how to send them away.

Being a Catholic country, dabblers of the Spirit of the Glass are supposed to recite the Apostle's Creed, the Our Father, the Hail Mary and the Glory Be first, before a Spirit of the Glass session. After saying goodbye to the spirits, they repeat the prayers again.

The "entity" whom just about everyone in the entire Philippine archipelago summoned, was Jose Rizal, the national hero. Duh.

☙

Papa and us kids did it once at home.

One time, a dog of ours died. We buried the dog in the back of the house, in the area where the old demolished mini slum apartments were, which our grandparents once rented out behind our big house.

The hole we dug revealed a square cemented block, which Papa said had always been there when his parents bought the property. All this time he had wondered what was hidden there. Mama said it looked like a septic tank, but Papa liked to think that the block probably hid Japanese treasure. He was playing with us kids.

We covered it back together with our dog, but we eventually had the idea to do a Spirit of the Glass session and ask what can be found under that square slab.

Using a permanent marker, we wrote the usual A-Z, 1-9, 0, Yes and No on the cartolina and got a drinking glass to invert and use as a pointer. "Goodbye" may also be written, but it was believed that the spirit had left once the glass stopped moving. We darkened the room and did our prayers. Then we asked for the spirit of our national hero to come to us to answer a few questions.

The glass moved as usual, but we freaked out so we said goodbye to our national hero, said the necessary prayers and we pretty much still did not know what was under that slab. Mama was in the kitchen and once again said it was just a septic tank.

We did not want to end up a little crazy like Papa's boss' daughter. We had a big house too. We cannot allow it to be haunted. That was the first and last session we did. Besides, when it started to move, we suspected it was Papa playing a trick on us.

I had never been curious this way. I had always believed the board was too creepy and unpredictably dangerous. What also discourages Filipinos from doing the Spirit of the Glass was the use of a drinking glass as pointer. I heard that a drinking glass made of real glass should be used, not plastic nor anything else. If it unintentionally flew off the board, like in the movies, it would break. Broken glass is never fun to clean up. Mama hated breaking glass because she tended to be the one cleaning up.

☙

My doubts above reminds me of a legendary creature called *aswang*. This accursed human being, like the mythical werewolf, supposedly changes from human to monster during the full moon.

A special oil is supposedly spread on the body, and the person splits at the torso. Wings that look like a bat's enable the upper body to fly, to look for a victim, while the lower torso and legs stand on the ground.

Seriously, if this creature were real, there should be real pictures of it by now.

Not everything in the Philippines can be believed.

Well, just in case, if the aswang were true, it is said that if you happen to see a standing lower torso, you should pour sand or salt into the cavity. The aswang will die if it did not reconstitute itself before sunrise.

On the other hand, analyzing what supposedly happens related to the aswang is another story.

Aswangs supposedly like fetuses. Pregnant women supposedly wake up in the morning, with or without blood coming from their wombs and out through their sexual organs, but the babies they were carrying would be gone without a trace. I have never met anyone who claimed mysteriously losing a baby this way, but this sounds like the use of women for alien reproduction.

So alien abduction and atrocities might also be happening in the Philippines, just like nearby Australia, New Zealand and other Asian countries.

☙

Maybe, Ouija boards and Spirits of the Glass can be believed, but I tend to think that they are a no-no. Like I said, this chapter sounds like a good story, but I also go by my instincts. I don't endorse it.

I'm showing a similarity between the Philippines and the U.S. Not everything in the Philippines is exotic and foreign.

Chapter 11

An Encounter at the Path

I had a great aunt, whom I talked about in my other memoirs. She was my dad's aunt, his dad's sister. Theresa. We called her *Lola* Tesay ("teh-SAH-yee"). "Lola" means "grandma."

Her great accomplishment was that she too finished college in Manila, the only one who did amongst her siblings, at around 40, when Mama had already married Papa, which itself was also a late decision.

My parents met in college, when both ended up living in Manila to study in the same university. Mama was from another island, Bohol, and was sent to Manila for a college education. Papa wanted to become a lawyer, so marriage had to wait. For a while, Mama found a job in Manila, but she went back to Bohol, where Papa and his parents came to propose to Mama's family.

Mama's dad was a doctor, supposedly one of the first doctors on the island. The home where Mama grew up was a 3-story building. Her dad had, on the first floor of the building, a reception area, a medical office, an examination room and an operating room with an operating table. There were a few rooms with beds on the first floor. The second floor had even more rooms for patients. The third floor was the residence where the family lived. The house faced the town plaza. Most homes were one or two stories high. I guess Mama's family impressed Papa's parents, but when they realized that Mama was not bringing that prestige to Manila, they started to dislike her.

Back to my great aunt. Lola Tesay's college education did not equate to class either, nor did it change her crassness.

When us kids did something wrong, and we got shouted at or punished, she also had to have her say with us, using deep Filipino words equating to being the bastards from the Bible worthy of eternal damnation. Well, her favorite word was *suwail* ("soo-wah-EEL"), which meant "rebellious," and for it to come from her was uncalled for.

I never learned she finished college until around high school, but once in a while, she stayed with us in Manila. For the most part, she stayed on Lubang Island, tending to her farmland.

I thought Lubang Island was primitive, electricity was turned on for about 10 to 12 hours a day, from the morning during weekdays. The nights remained dark. I finally figured electricity must had been turned on only during work hours.

When I was in grade school, I only saw her as an old lady who liked to tell us stories of their ordeals during World War II, and liked to mention the word "suwail," complete with a bad facial expression.

Once, I needed help with a homework, she volunteered to help me, but she told me to write the word "superiors," meaning that I needed to listen to those who were older than I was. I refused to write it down, my point being that it was the first time I had heard of the word, and that my teacher might get the impression that my answer was just dictated to me by someone else. I probably implied at that time, and she probably got the impression, that I didn't trust her aptitude.

I don't know what happened to her when she was growing up, but she had a mannerism—a giggle or a laughter ended her comments. She also easily got terrified. She never liked to hear the word *multo*, which is Filipino for "ghost" or "entity." She did not like us playing with flashlights or lamps on the dark nights on Lubang Island, nor even during the blackouts in Manila, which usually happened during typhoons, when we held the lights by our chin so we looked scary, pretending to be multos.

☙

Filipino and English words. The English word, "boondocks," comes from the Filipino word, *bundok* ("boon-DOHK"). Everyone knows that. Americans coined the English word while in the Philippines. Filipinos have this bad word, *buwisit,* which comes from "bullshit," also invented when the Americans occupied the Philippines. I wonder about a couple more words though.

Lemuria and Atlantis supposedly disappeared off the face of the earth. Lemuria was supposedly in the Pacific.

The Filipino word for "ghost" is multo, which seems to have come from the Spanish word *monstruo* or the English word, "monster."

There is another word for ghost. *Mumu* ("MOO-moo"), and some say it is from the word Mu, which is short for Lemuria. It might also come from the word multo, because it is used to scare small kids from avoiding spots they should not go to.

Adults would tell kids, "Don't go there, there's a mumu over there."

☙

Back to Lola Tesay. In her defense, when we were on Lubang Island, I had seen her count lots of money. She had her own farmland and her own tenants. She placed her money in some homemade pouch in her homemade panties.

She finished college in her forties. Then she married a man, who was about twenty years older than her. This man, she claimed, was really just for companionship, because she told us she did not want to live alone, and that was understandable especially for someone like her.

She was married to *Lolo* Milio, or Grandpa Milio. Kuya Jing and I enjoyed visiting with them because he was educated. He hummed tunes to himself and twiddled with his fingers all the time. Once in a while, he stopped twiddling and shaped his gnarly, left knuckle up in the air while his gnarly right knuckle went to and fro, as if he were playing air violin. Then he went back to twiddling.

No he wasn't senile. He used to play the violin. He never complained of arthritis, but his fingers were bony. He had a collection of old vinyl records. Some of the vinyl had been visited by termites. His greatest attraction for Kuya Jing and I, was his huge collection of years and years of Reader's Digest magazines, which my brother and I enjoyed reading when we vacationed on the island.

Lubang Island had a main road. The pier, where the boats from Manila docked was located in Tilik, or Tilic, so Tilik was the Rome of the island. The municipality, or the main "city," still rural, was Lubang, which was about 10 kilometers, or 6 miles, away. To us kids, having been there when we were small, Lubang was a thousand kilometers away from Tilik. My family had trucks and Land Rovers at different points in time. We never imagined walking on that road. My grandparents had a house in Tilik. Lola Tesay's house was next door.

Lolo Milio had a house in the town of Lubang, but he lived and stayed the night with Lola Tesay in her house in Tilik. He walked each way, everyday, and that was his daily exercise. He did not have to work, I think he was a teacher and was retired. My grandparents did not like him, because they said Lola Tesay got nothing from him. He was just another mouth to feed. He had kids who didn't take care of him, some of whom lived in the United States.

To Lola Tesay, all that mattered was a companion, so she would not live in fear of invisible beings. If that to her was all that mattered, then Lolo Milio was everything to her. In retrospect, Lola Tesay probably came to Manila to stay with us when Lolo Milio had to be out of town himself.

In the late '80s, after the death of Lolo Milio, Lola Tesay and I came to Florida for a visit with Aunt Li, my dad's only sister. Lola Tesay talked proudly about her stepchildren, irritating me with talk of their successes, blah blah blah. She had their phone numbers. They lived in California and elsewhere. She finally attempted to call them, to say hello, and I was sure that in the back of her mind, she wanted to take a trip out of boring Florida, in Tampa, where my Aunt Li lived and worked and where we were supposed to stay for a few months. Lola Tesay got ahold of them, talked to them a few times, none of them invited her to visit.

Anyway, back to the Island of Lubang. In the late '70s, and this is really what would be so important, I can probably tell it to you in one or two sentences, but this is a memoir of sorts, after all. Lolo Milio was walking back to Tilik. It was the usual time, late afternoon, when the sun was no longer scorching hot.

Only one road connected the towns. Everyone called it the "Main Road." The main road followed the coastline, so it turned as the coastline turned.

There was this undesirable bush called, "aroma." Since aroma followed the coastline, it also followed the main road on the side of the sea. Sometimes it also grew on the other side of the road where the rice fields were. Aroma here, as I'm describing it, does not mean "smell." Aroma is a woody bush that has thorns that can grow past an inch.

During Holy Week, when penitents paraded on Lubang Island, hooded to hide their faces, flailing their backs with homemade whips made of young hollow bamboo dowels that made a haunting, rhythmic, musical noise, or carrying crosses,—some of them wore crowns of thorn made of this endemic aroma.

As Lolo Milio walked on the main road, some parts of which were unpaved, on the side, he saw a being, that looked like a baby, that was also as tall as a baby, scampering.

It was naked and the entire body was red in color, according to him. It ran backwards, not forwards. It seemed impossible for it to see its way, but it scurried adroitly, coming from behind him on the other side of the road, impossibly running backwards with ease, as if it knew where to go, and then it turned onto some dense aroma bushes a little further down and more to the side of the road. Where it made the turn, backwards, it went right smack into the aroma and disappeared!

When he told us this story, he swore to God that he wasn't lying. He said his heart pounded like he would have a heart attack.

He walked faster, panicked but did his best not to show it. He thought that if he let the being know he saw it, or if he showed fear, the being might terrorize him some more and follow him home to Lola Tesay's house.

I guess, I'm assuming that most of my readers would not be Filipino. I'm painting a picture of where my family lived. The supernatural happens there as well, told and interpreted by the locals.

Chapter 12

Intro-Version

I became introverted, no thanks to childhood. Having to keep a secret, such as incidents of molestation and more, being secretly gay, feeling less favored by Papa on certain occasions. I mentioned all this in my other book, **Wonder.**

The next shock of my life was when the school changed it's practice of grouping the classes according to our grades, what they called homogeneous or in this case, "homogenius" sectioning, to heterogeneous, or "heterogenius" sectioning.

I struggled with my grades in Grade 6. We had a Grade 7 level, but we also had an acceleration program. If we made the cutoff grade, we got accelerated.

My brother had no problems with acceleration. He had been Valedictorian from Grade 1. He "lagged" in Grade 6, becoming rebellious. In the end, he placed second, Salutatorian. Becoming Salutatorian was rebellion to him. He passed classes with high grades with eyes closed. His literary compositions were read in class. I wished I was a better writer. I am now, I guess, as long as he makes no attempts.

Throughout that year, I was told that it was okay to lag behind, and not to make the grade for acceleration. It was okay for me to do Grade 7, while my brother entered the next building across the street.

I refused. I got used to having my brother as a classmate.

There was a time when my brother got in trouble, he was not in class then, I was.

A classmate, as he was explaining whatever trouble that was to the teacher, pointed at me and said, "You can ask his brother, Val, over there."

My teacher, in my defense, turned to me and took the opportunity to say, "Do you know what you should say, Val, whenever this comes up? You should say, 'Am I my brother's keeper?'"

I told her I did not understand what she meant.

She said that's what Cain told God when God was looking for Abel.

I felt safe in my brother's shadow. Whatever he did that time, I shut it out. One time he got in trouble for selling peanuts which was harvested when Papa tried farming on Lubang Island. He got in trouble another time, when he sold mimeographed copies of a form which my classmates were supposed to handwrite.

I was stressed to make the grade because no one was encouraging. I eventually made the exact average grade for me to be accelerated to high school, just like my brother.

To my surprise, they separated us. Years later, I was told that they intentionally did that over the next 3 years of our high school life, because I seemed to need to get away from my brother's shadow. Duh. They thought it was a good experiment. It was not.

What they did not take into consideration was that the less intelligent ones, the students who were larger, older and more mature-looking, because they went through Grade 7, were mixed in with me. I was bullied in high school over the next 3 years because they saw me as a bully's victim. My introverted demeanor was too obvious.

I also had a large forehead. Even when I was small, it was obvious. They teased me about that as well.

I suppose I talked with a lisp sometimes. The bullies teased me about that.

It was then that I learned to count my blessings. I also counted how many more days to go before school was out.

There was a public elementary school across the street from my school. The students went to school with less books in hand

and some wore thong slippers. We had always been seated in class alphabetically. I always ended up in the back and towards the window. I looked out once in a while, I see those children. I reminded myself that I was lucky enough.

Comic books became my escape, I eventually had 3 boxes by the time high school was over. They were my escape. By then I promised myself I would one day visit New York and check out where the comic book offices were. Needless to say, I discovered they were not Disney World-like edifices the way I envisioned them, but that was years later. Back to my nightmarish high school life.

I became more religious in high school. My school was a Catholic school, run by the Capuchin Order, which was started by St. Francis of Assisi. The school had a big church, or the church had a big school. I went there with another friend, almost everyday. Luke and I hung out from Grade 3. He was also Section A. We went to bookstores, where he confidently stole paperbacks.

He told me he went to church everyday, sometimes during lunchtime, sometimes after school hours, and so I went with him a few times.

I got so bullied in school one day, on my third year, that I punched one of the bullies, and then cried in class. The main bully was still amused, happy and delighted. His smile never left his face. On that fateful afternoon, I went to church. I faced the statue of the Lady of Lourdes, and asked for help.

In less than a week, one day, the main bully was absent. The counselor came up to our class. He said the guy would not be here for a while, because his dad died of a massive heart attack. The bully, it turned out, had been rebellious at home as well, and he had an argument with his dad. The guy blamed himself for his dad's death.

The counselor told us that his grades were failing anyway, and so it was decided that he would take a break from school. He was to come back next year to repeat this same year level.

I can't blame the counselors through the years for not coming to my aid. I wasn't talking about my own problems to anyone but God.

The bullying stopped, I got my usual good grades. By the fourth year, there was a new experiment. This time they were attempting to save their reputation of being a school that produced smart students.

They said mixing intelligences did not really influence and improve the less smarter ones, it only made the grades of the smarter ones suffer.

The school worried about their own prestige, that no thanks to their heterogenius sectioning, our batch might not have as many people entering the top colleges, especially the strictest, most challenging university, the University of the Philippines. So for our senior year, they finally regrouped the smartest students into one class. I was once again paired up with my brother. My best friend Luke did not make the class.

I saw the bully back in school, repeating junior year. Guess what. I had grown taller. The guy looked shorter.

My brother, myself, and a good number of my classmates during that senior year met up again at the University of the Philippines.

I'm in my late forties now. I still have my large forehead. I still have my hair, which I grow past shoulder length. I get haircuts once every 8 months to a year and a half. I like looking haggard in my long hair. I celebrate it.

I'm out, gay, and writing memoirs from the perspective of an artist. I still act straight although my latest art thing to do was making porcelain dolls. I think my doll art is akin to male chefs in restaurants. You get past a point of excellence and gender and stereotyping stop to matter.

I am still religious, and keep to my own version of the Golden Mean, although I do have my outbursts of anger and frustration.

I had connected with my former bullies on the online social

networks. I hope we all became better human beings. Some of my former classmates, the ones with the nice hair and hairlines, some of whom were my bullies, have lost their hair.

I am, like my distant cousin, Liwanag, whose beautiful face and light, fair skin I still remember, with her long, flowing hair, an immortal goddess, I mean, god.

Chapter 13

College, Speedreading & the Girl

In grade school, whenever my brother was praised in class for his English compositions in English class, or for his Filipino compositions in Filipino class, I wished I wrote like him.

While in college, I saw the movie, *Bladerunner,* in the theater with a friend of mine, as soon as my brother told me it was good. He saw it the week before, probably with his girlfriend at the time.

There was a phrase in the movie, something like, "The light that burns twice as bright burns half as long."

This made me think to pace myself. I liked to read. I had extra books on vocabulary. I read the melodrama of American comic books.

I felt my brother was winding down a little. He did not care too much for high grades anymore. He still got higher grades though. We still made it to the University of the Philippines. We both chose pre-medicine, but we both decided not to pursue medicine. We continued to become classmates in some classes.

My dad, through the years, did not consider himself successful. He worked for the BIR, the Bureau of Internal Revenue, the IRS version of the Philippines, for many years. He then got connected and worked for the president of the Republic of Palau. Palau was an American territory. They used dollars and I guess it was as privileged as the US Virgin Islands and Puerto Rico.

When I was in Grade 1, Papa paid my music teacher for extra time for me to start playing the piano. In other years, he took the three of us, Kuya Jing, Dinna and myself to the Yamaha School of Music, located at a mall, every Saturday, where we learned to play the keyboard.

He also took my brother an I every Sunday to Manong Boy. *Manong* ("mah-NOHNG") means "older brother" in Cebuano, Mama's language, spoken in Bohol, Cebu and some other islands or parts of islands from the middle of the Philippines to the southern parts. It is the second most popular language. "Boy" is a nickname. I think his real name is Eduardo. He's an older, distant relative of Mama. They don't use "Kuya" on the middle islands of the Philippines.

There was a weekday noontime live variety show in Manila which we watched as often as we can whenever school was out. Our parents learned that Manong Boy was the band leader of the show. We saw him for a second or two whenever the camera panned to his band, just as he was doing that 1-2-3-4 count with his hand and his head. It turned out that he lived nearby. He agreed to teach me bass guitar, and my brother lead guitar.

Papa also paid for my brother and I to learn arnis on Saturdays when we were in grade school. Arnis is more known now as eskrima or kali, the martial art that used a pair of sticks.

Throughout those years, I had the notion that I played second fiddle to my brother. Especially the bass guitar lessons to his lead guitar lessons. In hindsight, I owe my dad a lot.

If there was anything he should have done, he should have explained to me what the motivation or motivations were behind all these extracurricular activities.

In the U.S., I volunteered in theater for many years. Nowadays, it's so easy to ask, "What's my motivation?" I think, if there was anything that Papa missed, he missed explaining to me the importance of the bass guitar. He never took us to a concert. He nor Mama never explained to me why I had to face a piano or a keyboard. If he found a way to make me find my motivation, I would have been a much better musician by now.

By college, he sent us to what I considered the most magical, most exciting extracurricular activity. He sent us to speedreading school. It was then that I suddenly got better at writing. My compositions for the Filipino and English classes, in college, finally got read in class. I got A's.

Years later, I Googled the Filipino literature professor I had. It turned out that this mustachioed man, who read to the class "great writing by this classmate of yours, who will not be identified"—my works—this man was a legendary, award-winning writer himself.

Papa's speedreading workshop paid off. Something in my brain was unleashed.

I got disinterested in pursuing Medicine. I wanted to shift to Business. Papa and I had our violent disagreements. Mama told me to just finish my bachelors and proceed with a masters soon enough, as opposed to shifting and spending the same amount of time in school, and still only ending up with a bachelors degree. She made sense.

*

Back to Mama. During those college years, I don't know how I ended up with Mama again. This time, on a Saturday, she took me to a faith healing gathering.

What I noticed there, was that the lower ranking faith healers had a few strange practices.

They held the left and right pinkies of the "patients," placed them side by side, and compared them to see if their lengths were the same.

Mama asked, and I heard them explain, that if the little fingers were not of the same length, it can be a sign of possession or evil influence. Mama smiled. I looked at her. I did not think she bought the explanation, but she was great in hiding her incredulity.

I too thought it was a stupid notion. We could be wrong.

I saw this girl whose demeanor seemed like she came from a rich family. However, she wore a long-sleeved shirt. I ended up next to her, so we talked.

She showed me rashes on her arms. More were on her neck.

She said it was all over her body. That was why she was there, to be healed because doctors had not been able to heal her. Years later, here in America, through the internet, I figured her condition was a really bad case of psoriasis. We discovered we were going to the same university.

I eventually saw her a few times at the university, hanging out with her friends, wearing long sleeves. One day, I finally got the courage to approach her. I said hello and identified myself as the guy at the faith healers. I asked if she remembered me.

She was cold and aloof. She seemed to want me to go away. I thought I understood her.

There she was, a student, very social, looking upper class, with peers who behaved like her. She made a gesture of whispering to a girlfriend, while looking at me. Then the other girl laughed a little.

I got the hint. I went away and never bothered her again. I'm sure she still had her rashes. I wondered if she told her friends that she tried faith healing. Faith healing was a thing for the masses, not for the upper class. Maybe she was not ready to face something. She was ashamed of something.

Chapter 14

An Incomplete Grade

College was supposed to be four years. Mine and my brother's took five. From this point on, let me state my excuses, I mean my reasons, for the delay.

My brother's main excuse was that he "probably" did not want to become a doctor anymore. I felt the same way. I wanted to become a writer, but I couldn't tell anyone that. I was also interested in Business and Economics. I didn't want to become an artist yet, although I'd had my bouts with art as I grew up. Art supplies in the Philippines were expensive. There was a graphic arts supply store nearby, where we lived. It was one jeepney away. I only bought tech pens.

My last writing hurrah was an English term paper. On that fourth year.

The teacher said, "Most of you guys in this class are graduating pre-medical students. You already have difficult science classes and I know you need to make the grade, so I'm grouping you for the term paper project."

I was grouped with my friends, my batch mates, but as we were discussing what topic to do, I had a disagreement with one of them. My disposition was bad, I made her feel my wrath. I actually made her cry days later, and for the life of me, today, I still feel remorse for that incident, but I can no longer recall the reason for our disagreement.

I can remember the frustration that I was going to overstay by a semester anyway, because I failed a few classes through the years and I was unable to catch up, even though I did some summer semesters.

I eased out of the term paper group.

I approached my teacher, and asked for a grade of "Incomplete." I told her I wanted to become a writer, and this term paper would be an opportunity to train myself to write something that would be very impactful and important to me.

An incomplete grade, an "INC," on the temporary transcript gives the student a full year—two regular semesters and a summer semester—to complete the requirements for the class. All the grades from that class remained valid for the duration. If the reason for the incomplete got completed during the year, the final grade got issued, calculated from all the requirements and grades, as if the lapse in time never happened. If the reason for the incomplete never got completed, the INC becomes a failing grade, a "5" in my school. This meant that the class, had to be retaken.

Regular grades went from 1, the highest, to 3, a passing grade with increments of .25 in between. After the 3 is a 4. This is a conditional grade, where the student usually needs to retake some sort of comprehensive exam. If passed, the 4 gets upgraded to a 3. Sometimes, the class can be retaken, and the 4 gets erased from the transcript, replaced by the final grade of that next try. 5 is a fail, permanently recorded on the transcript. The student will have to retake the class again, but the 5 remains on the transcript.

She gave me all the time in the world to decide what topic I wanted to do for my term paper.

Around that time, I liked reading books and articles on the paranormal. On dwarves and other invisible entities. I saw a couple of books on psychic surgeons at the bookstore. I had wanted to become a writer. My subject: the paranormal.

A great title for my first envisioned worldwide bestselling book occurred to me. ***Psychic Philippines.*** I thought it was a neat title, playing with the letter "P" and the way it was pronounced. I thought each chapter will tackle strange paranormal events happening in the Philippines.

One of my science classes required us to do field work. We were required to go to a province, research, and write a scientific paper about something related to the place.

We wrote about the dangers of the Bataan Nuclear Power Plant, which was nearing completion, but which the residents do not want. It had already cost the government $2.3 billion dollars and it was going to use atomic fuel.

I was the one who suggested to my group where to go and what to tackle. I did not really care about the topic. It was really because I had relatives there. We did not have to worry about where to stay overnight.

That night, with the interview for our schoolwork over, we got into talking about the paranormal. We were in Mariveles, Bataan, which was part of the World War II Bataan Death March.

Someone said, that after the Liberation, after the surrender of the Japanese, and the American soldiers were freed, the American soldiers were bathing in Balon Anito, a secluded, more rural spot, a little farther from the town of Mariveles, where they stayed. *Balon* means "well" or "water source." *Anito* means "enchanted beings" or "enchanted idol."

The bathers spotted what was locally known as a *kapre,* a very dark-skinned gigantic ogre, with piercing red eyes, known to smoke a large rolled tobacco while sitting on a tree branch. The kapre was indeed sitting on a tree branch, smoking, just like the legend, naked, just like the bathing soldiers.

The soldiers, frightened, ran back to town, all naked.

Our interviewees said this was a true story. More strange events had happened in Balon Anito. Balon Anito was worth revisiting if I had the guts, but, dealing with unknown, nonhuman entities, I didn't think it would be for me.

☙

I don't think *Psychic Philippines* will ever be realized. The reasons, my reasons, don't stem from my inner conflicts.

In the U.S., based on the radio shows which talk about the

paranormal and UFOs, every guest specializes on a topic. They spend their lives chasing their weird, unexplainable topic, and a good number of them, to date, still cannot produce valid proof. When they need to go somewhere relevant, they just hop on a plane or their car. There's always a hotel or motel nearby.

The Philippines is a network of islands. There is geographic separation, language barriers, and less than ideal accommodations. You cannot dial 911 for emergencies. Such a smaller place than the U.S. has just as many legends and myths.

It would be smart to concentrate on one area or topic of interest.

※

Back to my English term paper. I went to her office to give her my idea for a term paper, worthy of submission after a year of research and field work.

My "field work," this time was in Manila. Convenient. The trips were hour-long jeepney rides. I still had the safety of home. No need to meet elusive, enchanted, legendary beings. A topic that would be great for someone who had been questioning going to traditional medical school.

My paper was to be about the Filipino psychic surgeons.

Chapter 15

Activism

I went to the University of the Philippines for a Bachelor of Science degree in Biology.

It's a 4-year degree. I guess I had so much fun because I finished in 5 years. Kuya Jing did as well.

The year was 1986. Then President Ferdinand Marcos got ousted by the People Power Revolution in February. We started the semester in November 1985, classes got suspended certain days, the president and his family went to Hawaii, we came back to school to finish college. School was out by March, as usual.

I was no longer going to school except that I had to submit my English term paper about the psychic surgeons. I was able to submit it in March, so I was obviously busy and tense with that term paper, that I didn't care about any revolutions. The demonstrations affected me the semester before that, from June to October 1985. I had a few classes left and I was already overstaying by a semester. My brother was also overstaying, but he didn't seem to care.

I admired my brother. He drove a Land Rover to school, he made excuses to our parents to get himself and I home later than expected, so he can be one of the university's Red Cross volunteers during the demonstrations. We had an agreement that we would go home together, as if we were busy with schoolwork. Two students using the Rover, being studious, sounded better than him coming home alone with stories about the riots. One crucial, violent day, my brother talked about hearing the whiz of bullets as the opposing parties exchanged fire. One of his friends, another student from the university, got hit by a bullet within that week, and my brother was the one who took him to the hospital.

Not counting that bad incident, which happened toward the end of that semester, I didn't worry too much. I was actually a little irritated by his extracurricular activity, because when he started mentioning names of schoolmates I did not know, or greeting students I no longer recognized from any possible Biology courses that we were both doing, I got the feeling that he was socializing too much.

I think, as a universal rule, not just in the Philippines, if you get into activism or on the fringe of society, you shared ideas and ideals with people who felt the same way. Over beer. Over whisky. Over a jug of soda mixed with vodka, whisky, or beer or all of the above.

One time I was with him drinking with our mutual friends. There were 5 or 6 of us. We had a jug that had a spout. My brother and a few friends expertly mixed two different soda bottles, juice, and two types of liquor. One was cheap local gin. The result was a dirty brown concoction. We enjoyed the drink, then we all rode the Rover and headed home.

As usual, whoever was on the Rover got taken home. My brother was generous that way. We were university students, mostly from the same high school, so we lived around the same section of Manila.

My brother felt like throwing up. He said, "I need to stop to do a 'blow-by.'" He said that sentence in Filipino, but that word "blow-by" was in English; that's not a translation. The phrase, or word, came out of his mouth like it was a normal phrase.

As soon as he stopped the Rover, got out, and threw up by the side of the road, I understood what it meant. I figured that was what he did as I waited in the library for my ride home, maybe every single time. As I waited and waited and waited up until late at night waiting for my ride at the botany-biology pavilion's library run by the biology student association of which he and I were members of. He must had been "mixing" socially with his activist friends.

I had never heard of it until then, but it was obvious that he had said it before, just as normally as he mixed the drink we had that late afternoon, just a little off the university, in the scenic, hilly, fresh air, open space, grassy area, towards where the university housed their employees and teachers.

Well, back then I worried about my brother. That's why remember this, I can remember who drank with us, but our group always hung out anyway. Not that I'm being too square about the drinking part. Now, I'm a writer. Writers tend to be sensitive to word use.

In 2002, I went to bartending school. I learned to mix drinks. Now my brother and I can both mix drinks!

☙

Writing to me, now, and now that I'm older, especially this book on the incredible things the psychic surgeon did and told me, *is* a form of activism. Even my brother just might get irritated from it. I have not lied about the details in the book. This is why I have included seemingly trivial, less exciting events. I'm also glad I was not in the middle of every story I have told. Sometimes, the experience of hearing a story is good enough, especially if it's strange. Well, I can safely say that every word I type is a true claim.

This must be my karma of sorts. I only participated a few times in rallies because I was worried about my grades. I saved my activist spirit for now, decades later. Now I put myself in the middle of attention, by being an artist and a writer.

I do care enough to debunk my own weird experiences and stories. After all, my bachelors degree was Biology. I later got into a masters in a discipline of Mathematics, Actuarial Science, just before I decided I wanted to become an artist.

These stories and my perspectives are my attempts to show that this memoir of sorts did not happen overnight. I am still letting you know that other than my shocking, yet objective, factual claim that I had seen psychic surgery, I still have my doubts about it and the other seemingly strange events, stories or claims that have come across me.

It's funny, but it was a challenge to proceed with this spiritual/paranormal memoir while debunking events and trying to be objective as I moved along.

My goal has been to write a memoir, a collection of related stories. I finally chose to write something about the strange. I can sensationalize it, embellish the events, lie if it would enhance the story, but I cannot. I have enough to write an honest, albeit less sensational book. My goal, of simply writing a book has been reached, and that's good enough for me.

I should still expect opposition. Karma. I should have volunteered way back with my brother. In my mind since preschool, I thought we were supposed to be inseparable. Except that he had stories of the sound of bullets passing by him coming from opposing forces. And the Land Rover.

What should be fun, and I should expect fun as well, as I expose myself through writing, is that this is writing on the fringe of the paranormal. I will attract people who entertain this.

If you are reading this, and you find something good for you to use, and you feel that you're with me on my level, or maybe if you're still a young kid into all this, when you eventually get to my level and older, we can be like my brother.

We'll have a drink and talk about our activism, whatever that is. The paranormal, the arts, LGBT issues, religious issues.

In case we meet and I'm with my brother, shake his hand and tell him you've heard good, inspiring, life-changing things about him from my books.

If you, Kuya Jing and I happen to be at someone's home, wherever that may be, you have a choice of who can mix you a drink.

Chapter 16

Star People

In the late '80s, in the Philippines, I discovered a paperback, *The Star People,* written by Brad and Francie Steiger.

It talked about people who fit a profile of physical attributes, beliefs and experiences in life, with the conclusion that perhaps they were seeded or placed here on earth to change it for the better.

Of course, that was a paranormal book. I read the book and had this willingness to believe it, especially because I was seeking to get over many bad past experiences, seeking to better myself, trying to find an alternative to pursuing medicine and feeling that I had a great mission to change the world.

I believed that I was one of those "Star People," because I was sickly when I was a child, my joints constantly ached, ever since childhood, I had a traumatic childhood, and once in a while I thought it would be nice for a flying contraption, like a UFO, to come pick me up just to travel elsewhere for a while.

My thoughts that a book was written by authors who bothered, and that it had international distribution, meant that I was not alone after all. There might be more people out there like me.

This was one element, one tiny sliver of a reason, this thought that there were more like me, that made me want to come to the U.S. around that time. To discover and meet people who were like me. Since the book was published in the U.S., there must be a lot of us star people out there in the U.S.

So Brad and Francie Steiger did make a huge impact on me. Their book made me feel better about myself, and my mental and emotional struggles eased up a lot. It was the book I needed to read.

☙

I eased off of my complaints about Papa showing favorites when I started to entertain the thought that although my parents were my biological parents, I may have come from another world.

☙

By the time I left home, however, my thinking changed again. I had come to believe that my mission, whatever it may be, details, was dictated and guided by God. Therefore, in my mind, I told myself, I had no other choice but to follow God's dictates. God had told me to become an artist and a writer. What a great excuse. Everytime my dad brought up my nonsuccess, I extrapolated on God's dictates.

By 1999-2000, as the internet improved and more websites went up, I discovered that there definitely were a lot of people who believed that they were "star people," as described by Brad and Francie Steiger.

☙

In the late '90s, I discovered the ABA, the American Booksellers Association, and that their annual convention of publishers, authors and booksellers had been held in Chicago for sometime.

By then, I already had a few brushes with publishing. I had a column for a free monthly paper, and I had also done some projects for HIV/AIDS awareness. Also, in the late '80s, I signed with a literary agent to get an art book, about making greeting cards using melted crayons, published, although we never got a publisher. I felt it was good to check out the book convention.

I lined up for registration on Day 1. I had my business cards. I also had a press pass representing the monthly paper and another set of credentials for a magazine I had been planning to get off the ground in a few months.

There was a lady who was checking everyone's credentials to facilitate a speedy registration process. She looked at mine.

She said, "Are you with the press?"

"Yes," I answered.

"Well, you're not supposed to be here," she said.

"What? I got my credentials and I have the money to register. This is my first ever convention," I said.

"No, I mean you're not supposed to be in this line. This is for people who are not part of the press. Yours is upstairs. There's no need to pay for registration for the press," she said laughing.

"I just go up to there?" I asked pointing.

"Yes," she said telling me what room I should go to.

I thanked her. I went up. I saw the press room. I registered. There were no lines. The press room was special. I felt like a VIP. They had free coffee and danish. They had press packets from publishers, hoping to get their books publicized. I served myself some coffee and had some food. I sat down for a while and let all this sink in. The press room was quiet but blood was in my head. I felt the forceful pounding of my heart. Clean, smart-looking press packets! It felt like I was in heaven.

સ

Looking at the schedules and appearances by authors, I discovered that Brad Steiger was going to be at the convention at an appointed time and place, to autograph and give away a new book that was coming out in the fall. I was excited and it felt as if God directed me to finally meet him in person. I thought that this was a chance to talk to him for a while and ask him about the Star People book.

I went on that fateful hour at the spot where he was going to be. I lined up. The line was not too long. I made sure I got a book from him.

The autographing section at the convention floor had a row of about 40 tables. There were retractable-belt crowd control stanchions in place assigned to each table so the convention attendees lined up in an orderly fashion. The way the hundreds of authors were scheduled for that 5-day convention, an empty table was in between each author present, so at every given time, there were about 20-30 authors actively signing and giving away their books. As the line of autograph seekers waned for some, new authors sat down next to them.

I went up to Mr. Steiger. Behind him, and to the left about 4 feet away, relaxing, was a lady. She must be his wife, I thought, because they both wore western outfits and they both seemed well-tanned. Brad Steiger wore a cowboy hat. The way he dressed, he looked like a personality—a celebrity in his own right, an author known mostly for his name on a book cover, who on certain occasions like that autographing day, dressed up to look good in public. Another lady who seemed to represent his publishing company, assisted him by taking the books from the boxes and opening them to the title page, where he can sign.

I never bothered to research about him, and what he had been up to all these years. It was the '90s. The internet was not too comprehensive yet.

He and I greeted each other. I got my book signed, "To Val," and then I walked away.

It was very anticlimactic, but I was happy. I realized that his book had changed and improved me at a time when I needed to. I had moved on. His book was good enough.

☙

What he and the other authors had conveyed to me, on that first year that I started to attend the annual convention on the business of books, was that anyone can become an author.

On that day of the convention, I was thankful I lived in Chicago. Some people, like Mr. Steiger and that lady, had to come from elsewhere to be there. All I needed to do was hop on the public bus, the CTA, the Chicago Transit Authority bus.

On the next year, I got the courage to hop on the free shuttle buses that picked up and dropped off attendees between designated hotel stops and the magical convention center. I just needed to dress like I was a serious attendee, which I was.

There was something else that impacted on me about Brad Steiger that day. I smelled alcohol on his breath. Maybe that wasn't a tan on him and the lady. Maybe they had more than one drink. It made me think that these authors are human beings too, just like me.

I will one day become published, I told myself. I will attend more publishers conventions just like this one, have plane reservations and stay in hotels. I'll dress up right, and sign my books. Maybe, while waiting for my scheduled time to show up for a book signing, I'll have a drink or two, or maybe have lunch first and have a drink on the side.

Some years ago, I Googled Brad and Francie Steiger. I guess they had separated. I got the inkling that they probably equally owned the franchise to the idea of star people. Since they can no longer work together, the idea stopped at that book that I read years ago. Life goes on. The lady he was with was his new wife.

Maybe one day I'll meet Brad Steiger again. We'll have lunch and I'll ask him what he likes to drink.

CHAPTER 17

THE PRAYER CONTINUES

When I was young, while on a plane to the U.S., uncertain of my future, just having graduated from college, I closed my eyes.

I visualized God, and told Him that from that point on, until I finally found my mission and achieved success and financial stability, my entire life would become one single prayer.

Years later, right now, I remember that "vow." I'm still within that single prayer, and in as many times as I have thought that I probably should say "Amen" to end it, I have not.

Well, there's nothing really great about this, if you ask me. I had come to accept this state of prayer, including my sins and bad thoughts that "may" have occurred during this process, as a given. Besides, I don't think I've achieved success, recognition and financial stability yet.

I'm writing this while still within that one single prayer that has yet to hear an "Amen."

The prayer continues.

Chapter 18

Superman & Other Thoughts

There was a busy commercial street in Manila that was my favorite haunt. It's not like a mall where everything is comfortable. It's a really busy street, a lot of cars, jeepneys and buses, traffic congestion, pollution from the exhaust, and pedestrians on the tiled sidewalk.

It's not a rich person's escape, but it's Manila at its most overburdened state, and it's a fixture. Avenida Rizal. Rizal Avenue.

This was in the '70s. What I liked about it was that there were about 3 bookstores in the area. Mama liked going there for school supplies before the start of the school year. My friend Luke also liked going there because of the bookstores. We went there together. It was in one of the bookstores that he swiped a book, a juvenile book either about rocks or butterflies and moths, lightning fast, followed by the run-walk to the exit door.

Avenida Rizal was where my beloved comic book sources were. On the sidewalks, at regular intervals were kiosks where imported American magazines were sold.

The lowest planks had piles of comic books, the cheapest of which had their covers torn off. The more expensive ones still had covers on them. I later learned that the covers were torn off because they got sent back to the distributors as proof of how many copies did not sell.

I think they came from the American bases, Clark Air Base and Subic Naval Base.

I started buying comic books here in 1976. To give you an idea of my time frame, the first Superman movie, with Christopher Reeve, came out about two years later in 1978.

1978. So there I was squatting and perusing, looking for comic books I wanted to read. Charlton Comics, Gold Key, Dell, those companies were still around.

I looked up, and I saw a paperback, *Last Son of Krypton,* by Elliot Maggin, whom I recognized as a DC Comics contributor. Seeing a paperback about Superman, I got excited. I knew I had read some of Maggin's comic book writings. Maybe I'll try to read this Superman novel, I thought. Being young, I had never read a comic book-based novel. I bought the book and some comic books, went home and started reading the novel.

There was an idea in the book that I never forgot, something of an adult nature.

It was Superman's thoughts, the consequences if he revealed his secret identity to the world. If everyone knew where Superman worked, where he lived and what his phone number was, people would be showing up at his office and his residence, his phone would ring incessantly, and girls would throw themselves at him. A lot of favors would be asked, people would pretend to be his friend. He was thankful he had a secret identity.

☙

In a way, what I want to convey here, is that after having seen with my own eyes and having proven that psychic surgery did happen, it's akin to having a superpower.

The psychic surgeon I met devoted himself to his cause of healing and spirituality. There was no backing out, unless he retired and closed his door to the needy which would had been a difficult choice. Even if he closed his doors, desperate people would be banging it, asking to be healed.

If he were in America, he probably had already been sued and ordered to stop practicing psychic surgery. The FDA would already had come after him. He might already had been prohibited from using the words "heal," "surgery" or "service."

Where he was, in the Philippines, he had to be consistent. He had to be there for his service, at his home every Sunday at 5 p.m.

It was not a regular job that can be forgotten after office hours. He had to be mindful of it 24/7, for days, making sure that he did not dissipate whatever psychic or religious energy he was tapping through physical, mental, spiritual and emotional strain, including sex.

⁂

There was an audiobook that I got ahold of in 1993. This lady claimed that she once died and went to heaven. That was the premise of the book she wrote.

She spoke of an announced, scheduled speaking engagement. It was held in an auditorium.

What surprised her was that the auditorium was packed. She said that it was then that she realized that so many people needed to hear her message.

When I heard her say that, I took it as a warning. This idea of healing is huge and overwhelming.

I can safely claim that I'm a writer and an artist.

I am not a healer. Eeks, did I just say that? Maybe I am? Oops. By denying, I probably am. Yikes. I hope I don't get overwhelmed.

The lady talked about an overwhelming number of people, in search of something. All she had was a message, and they all showed up.

What about my message? I tried to put myself in her shoes, and I imagined how things would have been different had she also really been able to heal. All this was a scary thought for me in 1993, listening to what the author had to say.

I was listening to Coast to Coast one time and this lady caller told the host, George Noory, that she died and came back. She discovered that she had healing powers, but she did not want it. She came across a sick person somewhere in public, and she felt compelled to come up to the person and "heal" the person. She told God, in her mind, no, she did not want to have the "power," and she did not want to come up to the person.

I think I'll worry about being overwhelmed another time. I'll just keep telling stories for now. It was my intention to tell stories that have a twist and a jerk somewhere towards the end.

※

At some Catholic churches in the Philippines, there are women, and sometimes men, dancing in front of the churches, by the entrance. They might be holding candles or flowers or something else. They're not disco queens, they usually just jiggle. They do their best. No one laughs at them. They're highly respected. They are part of the culture, tradition and religion.

People come up to these ladies, and I've also seen men dancing on occasion and they pay these ladies and men to dance to the Lord God for them, for their petitions to be granted. The women who pay the dancers usually have difficulty conceiving a child. Sometimes the request is for healing.

Does this work? Probably not, but it's in place. Do they believe it works? They probably do. It's probably like buying a lottery ticket. You don't get the chance to win if you don't buy one. What if it does work? It's all faith. It cannot be proven.

People pay for this mystical service.

The same would be the case for Rasputin. The family felt they needed him.

What if I wrote this book early on. What if Steve Jobs got it?

※

I should keep reminding you, the reader, that I still have my suspicions about psychic healing. I tell people that I believe all this is a combination of faith, placebo, hypnosis, autosuggestion, desperation for a positive result, and the fact that poor people are after solutions too, just like rich folks. Some people can afford to take trips anywhere in the world for some experimental drug or treatment. Majority can just take whatever they can that's just around the corner. Hmm, I'm thinking I might be there too, one of the options just around the corner and farthest towards the dead end alley. I wonder if I should probably be there for people.

The problem is that all this is unproven. Faith healing and fake healing both start with two similar letters, after which they diverge. So do hope and hoax.

☙

It's back to the 1978 book, *The Son of Krypton*, and Superman. We're not Superman. I'm not Superman. People might be desperate for help. Should we lift our psychic finger for them? There is no escape to a secret identity. The author Elliot S. Maggin's, or Superman's, thoughts of consequences stay with me.

Chapter 19

The Hotel

Two events. Actually three. Three people involved. This chapter is the first.

I was a bellboy for a few months. I wasn't happy. I liked my coworkers—the main doorman and all the other bell persons. Well, bellboy was the term I liked to use. I was in my early twenties. I felt younger calling myself a bellboy.

Okay, so I was a bell*man* at a downtown Chicago hotel.

When I quit and came back to say hello, one of the newer bellmen was a girl. She was young and beautiful, but I saw her work; she can carry huge suitcases. At that point, the hotel called all of them "bellpersons."

Let me give you a quick tour of the hotel as an employee. You cannot enter from the front. There was an employee entrance in the basement.

The hotel was situated somewhere in Chicago where the main entrance was on the upper street level, and the employee entrance was one floor below, on some sort of an underground concourse which connected with many other buildings in the area.

Most of the housekeeping department were female, and most of them were Hispanic. I took four semesters of Spanish in college, so I was glad to be able to speak some Spanish with my coworkers. They liked the novelty of being able to speak their language with a non-Hispanic person, although some Filipinos considered themselves Hispanic or Latino. I do have Spanish blood. A lot of people in Northern Spain has Papa's last name. The famed Spanish philosopher, Xavier Zubiri, looked like my grandparents and other distant relatives.

Mama's grandmother, my great-grandmother, was also supposedly pure Spanish. Plus many more of my ancestors were Spanish. I had been dyeing my hair black or brown black lately, but my real hair was lighter than brown black when I was small. My siblings and I are like Gregor Mendel's pea experiment. Kuya Jing and Dinna are darker skinned with black hair. Amelia and I are lighter skinned with lighter hair. I would much rather call myself Filipino. My eyes look Asian anyway.

Back to the hotel. We workers used the employee entrance at the concourse. Past the bundy clock were the locker rooms for men and women, where we changed into our hotel uniforms. Next to the locker rooms was the housekeeping window, where the attendants gave out or took back our uniforms. Behind this housekeeping window was a huge room, where the hotel guests' laundry was also done.

We got free food during lunch and free coffee during short breaks at the cafeteria.

This story is about the lady from the housekeeping window.

Almost everyday, I saw her during my shift. She was a Hispanic, middle-aged lady who spoke little English.

After my shift, I changed clothes in the locker room, and returned my uniform to her.

I understood the phrase, *"Que paso? Que paso?"* which meant, "What happened? What happened?"

Carrying luggage was a physical endeavor. Bellpeople always lost buttons and unraveled stitches. Whenever I showed her a missing button, or an unraveled area, she went into her usual, "Que paso? Que paso?"

With a smile, I answered back, *"No se,"* which meant "I don't know." That's Level 2 Spanish, which I had never heard from my non-Hispanic coworkers. Haha. All they knew were Level 1 Spanish. *"Hola!" "Buenos Dias!" "Buenas Noches!"* and *"Hasta Luego!"* That's why my Hispanic coworkers liked me more, I think, because I attended an extra day of Spanish lessons and knew five additional words.

Here is what is really important, and it really did not need all the fluff above to be conveyed to you.

One day, the lady came to work with her right arm in a cast.

So I asked her, "Que paso? Que paso?"

She spoke back in Spanish, which I understood. She told me she broke her arm and it really, really hurt. It happened at her home.

Having run out of Spanish words relevant to her incident, I reverted to English, asking her, "Would you like the pain to go away?"

She answered, *"Si, pero como?"* ("Yes, but how?")

I asked again, "Would you really like the pain to disappear?"

Once again, she said yes.

I said, "Our secret, okay?"

She smiled and nodded.

I did my hocus pocus. The exercises I will show you in this book.

She was amazed. The pain was gone. She asked me, "How you do that?"

I smiled and said, "Magic." I asked, "Does it still hurt?"

She said no.

I went to work. During my lunch break, I went back down to the cafeteria, passing by her window in the process. I asked how she was.

She said that the pain had gone away.

Everyday, from that point on, she kept telling me it never hurt again, always asking me how I did it.

I kept telling her, "Magic. I prayed over it."

In the next chapter, let me tell you about the next lady.

HOCUS POCUS LATELY

Chapter 20

The Cook at a Restaurant

Let me give you a taste of Filipino food.

A good number of Filipinos like to eat meat with white rice. Forget vegetables. Forget health. A good number, well, most Filipinos I know, will keep eating meat despite bad health conditions. Some really great tasting beef or pork entrees even have anchovies or salted brine shrimp, and Filipinos eat them, even if they had gout.

White rice is bland. The strong flavor comes from the entree, or dish. Filipinos like to use the word, "viand." It is the viand that has all the flavor, and because the flavor is concentrated, the bland, white rice is eaten with it. This is why Filipinos use spoons and forks, not forks and knives. The viand and rice are simultaneously placed on the spoon. Mmm. Yummy.

Here's another reason for the evolution of the spoon and fork. Because of the tropical weather, with a lot more tropical germs lurking, Filipinos and other tropical countries tended to slice, dice and mince their food more, and to cook their food longer, hence resulting in more soupy, softer and smaller food pieces, which no longer required the use of a knife.

There was a nearby Filipino eatery in Chicago, where for $5 dollars, you got two entrees and a cup of white rice. You go to the counter, tell the server you want the combo, the server scoops white rice on a Styrofoam plate, you point to two of the many already cooked entrees, or viands, they had on display, and the server scoops them into Styrofoam bowls.

The eatery salted the food more than the usual, I guess, because they were cooked in the morning in batches and had to keep all the way to the afternoon, maybe even the next day.

Whenever I ate there, I blended a sugar-free fruit shake from slices of about 5 to 8 frozen fruits which I kept in my freezer as soon as I got home. I didn't mind the bland taste of the fruit shake. This was my version of making amends with my body.

Since the Filipino community in Chicago is small, and since the place was nearby, the servers tended to become familiar with the faces of the customers. Familiar, friendly faces tended to get more food.

The workers, including the kitchen staff, also used the customer tables to sit down and eat during their own breaks.

One of the kitchen staff was this tall, slender Filipino lady who was probably in her early sixties. She was thin and very active. Whenever I went there with certain Filipino friends, we made sure we greeted her even when she was in the kitchen. We said goodbye to her after the meal, praising her cooking as usual. Whenever she was free, she came out of the kitchen to say hello to us. Of course, there were other workers in the kitchen, but she stood out, because she looked like everyone's relative who knew how to cook. She was someone you'll want to take charge in the kitchen when you're hosting a huge Filipino feast.

***

One day, I was with a friend. I saw her limping. She seemed to have trouble with her right knee. I asked what happened to her.

"Arthritis," she said. "It hurts and I have been limping for a few days now."

I smiled and said, "I can make it go away. It's a principle of hypnosis that I learned, so don't think I'm a psychic healer. I'm Filipino, but I'm not a healer. It's got something to do with hypnosis."

She said, "Okay. As long as the pain goes away. Do what you want."

I placed my right hand on her knee for about 20 seconds. Then I asked, "Does it still hurt?"

She walked around for a bit. She started to look astonished.

She asked, "How did you do that? The pain's gone!"

I laughed.

"I'm not limping anymore, see?" she added.

"It's hypnosis. I hypnotized you, but it's hard to explain," I said.

"Well, thanks!"

My friend and I went to the counter and ordered our food.

As we ate, she went back and forth between the kitchen and the dining area a few times. She no longer limped.

As my friend and I were leaving, I waved to her, and she hurriedly came up to me. Once again, she thanked me for the "healing."

I once again reminded her that it's something to do with hypnosis. I also reminded her that she still had to take her medications, whatever they may be.

About four months later, I was with the same friend when I went back for lunch. I saw her limping again.

I joked, "I thought I healed you. How come you're limping again?"

She answered, "Oh no, that was the right knee. Now it's my left knee that hurts. Arthritis again."

"Okay. You want the pain to go away?" I asked.

"I thought you would never ask. Go ahead. Do what you can," she said in a cheerful way.

So this time I placed a hand on her left knee. I probably did the same length of time, 20 seconds.

Then I asked, "How do you feel?"

Once again, she walked around. "How do you do that?" she asked, astonished. "The pain's gone again! I can walk around without limping! You've healed me again!"

I smiled and corrected her. "I told you it's hypnosis. I'm not a healer."

"So you just touch what aches and the pain goes away?" she asked.

"Yeah, but it doesn't always happen," I said.

"Well what if I approach you again because this aches?"

She pointed to her groin.

I laughed. I walked to where my friend was, by the food. We ordered and ate.

Once again, when I was leaving, she approached to thank me.

❦

I'd like to say that this chapter ends here, but I can't.

When I was in college, we had classes where we had to leave Manila, headed to an island or another province hours away from Manila, for field work. This meant that we had to stay somewhere. Good times. The nights were spent with fun jokes, sleight of hand magic tricks, long talks that made us bond more, and, usually, beer, and soda for the non-alcoholics.

One time, one of us performed playing card sleight of hand. Being that he was our equal, a fellow student, the magic was entertaining, but since he was not a professional Las Vegas performer, after the 10-minute duration of mysterious card tricks, we spent a good hour and a half bugging him to share with us the secrets behind the tricks he performed.

He had no choice but to oblige, or he would not have heard the end of it. So he kept repeating the tricks, until, one by one, all of us finally got it. That was fun.

❦

This magic trick I did with the lady seemed okay for those two visits that I was there.

On the third time that I was there for lunch, she and I said hi to each other. I asked about her pains. She said they never came back.

My friend and I sat and ate our lunch. She later sat with her coworkers for lunch about 2 tables away from us.

I overheard her telling her coworkers that I was a healer and that there are people in this world who have this power to heal.

⁓

A Las Vegas audience would have left the magician's theater astonished, entertained and satisfied. The performer would have been happy as well, counting his money all the way to the bank.

I'm not a magician, but I seemed to have done something. The lady *had* to share her experience with me with other people who probably didn't care about it.

I preferred that people not talk about me behind my back, especially when I ate.

But this was to be expected. It *is* in the nature of standing out.

I noticed that the succeeding times I went there for lunch, she seemed to have behaved with increasing seriousness about the mysterious topic that was me.

If you were me, would you still continue coming back to the same place for a quiet lunch?

Chapter 21

Aunt Li Getting Sick

Case #3: Aunt Li.

I had an aunt in Florida, Aunt Li, Papa's sister. In the late '80s, I stayed with her for a few months. This was the same time that I mentioned in an earlier chapter about Lola Tesay. This is Aunt Li's chapter.

It was just a year after I submitted my English term paper on psychic surgery, so that was also the time when I was in limbo about how I wanted to shape my future.

I guess Aunt Li was my first patient.

By the time Lola Tesay and I stayed with her, she was already okay. She recently had breast cancer and her breasts were removed. She underwent chemotherapy and radiation. She was flat-chested when at home, but she wore the supple silicone breast pieces whenever we went out.

I told her I wanted to pray over her while I was there, and I wanted to do it everyday when we got the chance. She agreed.

So I did my visualization hocus pocus everyday. That was all I did.

I never got any feedback from her.

Years later, her cancer came back, and my parents volunteered to stay with her to take care of her. I believe she did chemotherapy again.

Several months later, my parents left. I guess she got better.

Then in 2008, she sent for my sister Dinna to stay with her for a while. I guessed the cancer came back a third time. Maybe some telltale signs started again.

I never told my parents what my English term paper was for more than two decades. I thought it was useless to tell them. I never told my aunt I met this psychic surgeon who shared with me his methods from the first day he and I sat down, with pen and paper in hand. It was useless to tell anyone.

Dinna called me so many times from Florida, telling me she would not be able to last there. She did not want to stay there at all. In just a few days of being with Aunt Li, she wanted out.

I reminded her that Aunt Li probably really needed help. Dinna wasn't there for a visit. She was there to stay with Aunt Li for a while because she was sick.

Dinna insisted that Aunt Li was just fine and as healthy as she'll ever be.

I told Dinna that she had to stay there. She agreed to be there the moment she took Aunt Li's money for the plane fare. It cost money to fly from Manila to Florida and then back.

Dinna sternly said no. She was going to fly to Chicago to be with me, and then it's back to the Philippines for her.

In January, I applied for a "job." It was to volunteer to be used as a guinea pig, for a medical study of an experimental drug, which would had paid a good amount of money, but I got rejected because my uric acid, according to the CBC, the complete blood count, the blood report, was way too high. I was poor, depressed, worried, and probably affected by the winter. I can't even afford a bus pass and here was my sister who was jet-setting.

Dinna insisted to be with me when there was nothing I had to offer her. She insisted that we'll get by. She had no idea how bad my situation was. I kept telling her my situation. She would not have it.

Aunt Li let Dinna come to Chicago, after which Dinna changed her itinerary a few times again to get to Manila as soon as possible. I did not understand why she suddenly just wanted to go home. Dinna's stay with me lasted only a few days. We had an escalating altercation. She offered no reason as to why she suddenly wanted out and not stay with Aunt Li.

In my mind, Dinna was like a privileged, crowned Miss Firecracker ingrate in a small town festival who had the honor to light the long fuse. It was like she lit the fuse and walked away without even waiting to see nor looking back to see how wonderful the firecrackers lit up. While in Chicago, she called the airline are few times to get her trip back to Manila to a sooner and sooner date. Well, she said some nasty, bossy things to me as if she owned me. That got on my nerves, and so, in the middle of a February winter, I threw her out and she was forced to stay with an aunt, Papa's first degree cousin, for the rest of her stay in Chicago.

To this day, I feel guilty for what I did. My own sister, who came all the way from Manila, was rendered homeless in Chicago. We had since patched things up, but that was an expensive, nerve-wracking, emotional ordeal. I will gladly burn in hell for doing this to my sister. I deserve all the punishment that will be coming to me. We used to be buddies when we were growing up.

Obviously, February was months before December of that year. Aunt Li contacted her best friend of more than 40 years, Barbara, and they made plans to spend December in the Philippines, a trip they probably had talked about for decades. Barbara had never gone to the Philippines with Aunt Li.

I believe Barb still worked a regular job. Taking time off, especially to spend money and go halfway around the world, even for a week, serious plans needed to be made in advance. Barbara wasn't Filipino. She was an all-American white person, a very nice family friend, with no connection to the Philippines except that through Aunt Li, she had come to meet many members of our family through the years. I had met her, her kids and the rest of her family when I stayed with Aunt Li. We had picnics together.

By 2008, however, it had been a while since Barbara and Aunt Li had seen each other. They agreed to do the simplest thing—just meet at the airport hours before departure.

What a surprise for Barbara. Thinking they would just be vacationing, Barbara saw an unrecognizable Aunt Li on a wheelchair, frail as ever and her stomach, around her liver area, was bulging.

Just imagining the sight of my aunt, I'm sure no words needed to be exchanged to get Barbara to realize that she was taking her best friend back to the Philippines to die, never to be seen again.

Which was exactly what happened.

My frustration from this story was that while I was able to do my unproven hocus pocus on Aunt Li when I spent time with her in Florida, 25 years earlier, I wondered, what if I came back to visit again? I never found the time to return to her for a visit.

✧

I remember in high school, a teacher said something about Christ being hated by people in his own hometown. He said people also naturally find it difficult to listen to their own relatives. He said the same thing happens to preachers. A congregation of followers will listen before a relative does.

If I had a track record of healing, maybe my aunt would had valued a subsequent visit from me, except that I was the one who hesitated and did not want to get into psychic healing anyway.

✧

While still alive, staying in the Philippines, my aunt checked her emails. I read about cancer online. I sorted through possible cures and alternative therapies.

I felt I was guided to reading about this fruit tree called "graviola." Supposedly, its leaves and bark have properties that can eradicate cancer. It can be ordered online. The source of the tree was Brazil.

I searched for pictures of the tree and leaves. Pictures of the fruit came up as well. I stared at the pictures of the fruit, stared at them some more, and thought the graviola looked familiar. I read about the fruit. It was supposed to be sour-tasting. It looked similar to a Philippine fruit called "guyabano." I searched for the scientific names of these two fruits. They were the same! A possible alternative cure for cancer can be found in the Philippines.

It seemed to me that all my aunt needed to do was have her hosts, her youngest brother, Tito Pablo and his wife, both doctors, or Papa, to go get some guyabano leaves somewhere accessible so she can make tea from the leaves and drink it daily.

I emailed this information to her, including some links. A few days later, I got an email from her. Two words. "Thank you."

I also relayed the information to Papa, who was a few islands away, in Manila. He made it appear like it was hard work to find a tree so he can purchase a few leaves from the tree's owner.

I had finally started mentioning to some family members my experience with the psychic surgeon in 2007. This time, now that my aunt was back in the Philippines, I told Papa to look for the organization of healers. They should be easy to find because they would be in Manila. Decades had passed, I didn't think the psychic surgeon friend of mine was still alive. Having lived in the U.S. for so long, I had even forgotten his first name!

Well, I remember his first name now, but I still cannot remember his last name. I don't have any way to get in touch with him now. I won't be able to get his permission to reveal his name any time soon. I don't even know if he is still alive.

They all said that the option to search for a psychic healer won't even be discussed.

Aunt Li lasted a little more than a year before she passed away.

At the time that she died, I had just made some money. I volunteered to travel to Tampa and clean her house. Maybe the family needed someone to find some important papers in the house or whatever. They told me I was not needed.

While Aunt Li was still alive in the Philippines, I prayed for her to get better. I did some meditation and visualization exercises, seeing her as a healthy human being. I saw her coming back to her home in Tampa.

I guess what I tried to do for her did not work.

They had Aunt Li cremated. My uncle, Tito Pablo, took charge of whatever needed to be done in Florida.

In early 2013, before I started writing this chapter, I told Dinna once again about the psychic surgeon. I said I will email her a brief set of instructions on how the psychic surgeon prayed and visualized healing. I reminded her that I used the techniques on Aunt Li while I was with her.

She optimistically said, "Yeah, you did that and she lasted 25 years."

Honestly, I didn't agree with her. What I did may have helped, but there were a lot of factors that helped her live another 25 years. Dinna said that 25 more years after the first win over cancer was good enough.

But... if you, my beloved reader, choose to try the techniques, read on. I'm still saying, chances are, all this would not work, but I feel obligated to write about it.

All this is speculation, quite paranormal, unprovable, and I still take acetaminophen or ibuprofen for pain. I'm still just providing you with a good read.

☙

It is 2014. I finally learned why Dinna had to return to the Philippines. It's a long story, but she's not the ungrateful Miss Firecracker that I thought she was. Still, whatever she and I now choose to keep to ourselves, she should have let me know years ago.

Chapter 22

Hocus Pocus Lately

I had this temporary gig last year, 2013. There was this worker who sat on his high swivel chair, doing his job, but he was holding an ice pack on his left knee.

I approached him and asked him what was wrong with his knee. I was smiling. I thought I would do my hocus pocus on him as an experiment. It might work or it might not.

I asked him, "On a scale of 1 to 10, with 10 being intensely painful, how much pain are you in right now?"

He answered, "It's an 8 right now, but there are times when it's a 20, past 10 and very, very painful."

"What's wrong with it?" I asked.

"I got pins sticking in there." he said. He lifted his pant leg and showed me a knee with a few scars. "It's been operated on because of the pain, and now I got pins in there, and it continues to hurt everyday."

I said, "Okay, I'll make it go away. You tell me if the pain is gone."

I asked him to stand up. As I started to touch him, I said, "I'm gonna touch you at different parts of your body, and I'll make the pain go away."

I touched him on his knee, and then I said, "I need to touch you here, and then here, and then here..." I touched him on both his knees, on his shoulder, on his eyebrows, on the back of his knees, and I also touched him on the top of both his feet. I made sure I did not go back to his face and head after touching his feet.

Then I asked, "Okay, does it still hurt?"

"How did you do that? It doesn't hurt as much anymore!" he exclaimed.

I asked, "Okay, on a scale of 1 to 10, how much does it hurt now?"

"It's a 2."

I said, "Okay, I'm going to fine tune what I did, I'll bring it down to a 0."

I went to wash my hands in the sink and came back to him. I touched him a little more "seriously," in my mind, and went back to his cheek, his scalp and temple, his neck area, his shoulders, back to his knee, the feet, the back of the knee, his hand and forearm, and his knee again.

I asked him, "How does it feel now?"

"How did you do that? The pain's gone!"

"Are you in pain anywhere else?" I asked.

"I also have pins on my elbow. My elbow still hurts," he said, showing me his left elbow. I saw scars on his elbow as well.

"Okay, so we're done with your knee, I'll make the pain in your elbow go away," I said.

I touched him in places again.

I asked, "How do you feel now?"

He asked me again, "How did you do that?"

I laughed. "All pain is gone?"

"Yes, it's all gone! How did you do that?"

I thought it was funny, but I knew the dynamics of our relationship had changed.

Everyday that I saw him after that, I asked if his pain had returned. He said no. I made sure that I never conducted myself in a smart alecky way whenever I asked. I was concerned and I wanted to know, for his own good and for my own memoir, I mean, for my own good, if the pain came back.

He stopped looking at me as a normal person. I actually felt that I earned his respect. He made sure to say hello whenever he saw me.

About a week later, I told him to come up to me if he had any questions, because I was sure that his belief system might have changed and I wanted to make sure that he was okay when I leave the place, because my gig was almost over.

A couple of others saw me do it to the guy. One of them came up with a joke a day later, about bottling my tears so we can sell it on the internet.

I came back for another gig a couple of months later. The guy confirmed that the pain from both his elbow and knee had not returned.

I was with another writer on that return visit. I told him about what I did and that I was writing a memoir and including such events in it. I said he can ask the guy what I did.

The other writer later told me that the guy confirmed the healing, and added that he did not want to "jinx" it, and so that's why he had kept mum about it as much as possible.

Understandable. Yay, I got a chapter down. And this chapter's title will be the title of my memoir on healing: ***Hocus Pocus Lately.***

CHAPTER 23

NEGATRONS

In the chapter where I mentioned speedreading school, that school was actually a seminar situation that took place every Saturday morning. They said that our "official bible" was Richard Bach's *Jonathan Livingston Seagull,* because the main character, Jonathan, was into speed, and his pursuit led him to his incredible ascension into higher levels of being. You should read the book if you haven't yet.

In the book, there were other seagulls who were against Jonathan's quest to better himself. As he leveled up, he left more and more other seagulls behind. He tried to show the other seagulls what he was up to, and he pretty much got negative reactions from them. However, as the story progressed, he also met others who were on the succeeding higher levels he got himself into, and they were all very supportive.

ఞ

In the chapter where I mentioned that I seemingly hypnotized or maybe "healed" a cook at an eatery, I also mentioned that I came with the same friend on both occasions. I did not elaborate too much about that friend, but I will a little in this chapter. I had stopped talking to that "friend." I don't know if we will ever reconcile in the future, but even if we did, I'm sure we will conduct ourselves differently. For now, I'll just call my ex-friend "Carlos."

To make a long story short, Carlos had gout. I believe he still has it from time to time. I haven't talked to him in a long time, but I knew his eating habits and the increase in the dosage of his gout prescriptions through the years.

On the first time, Carlos saw me do my hocus pocus on the lady cook. He saw her limping and then he saw her walk normally without the limp. We bought our food from the counter, chose a table and ate. The lady sat nearby and continued to praise me. As Carlos and I ate, we joked and talked, as usual, except for what he had just seen. Carlos had nothing to tell me nor ask me about what I did. This happened again the second time the cook complained about her other foot. Carlos was with me again. There was no talk about my parlor trick.

Carlos was either uninterested, unimpressed or already adding more points to his disinterest or dislike in me. Maybe he was holding a grudge. He and I never talked about his problems. He like to keep his problems to himself.

Carlos had gout. He probably still does. I don't talk to him anymore. I had seen him walk with a limp a good number of times. Usually his gout attack was on his ankle joint on either his left or right foot. It inflamed and hurt for at least 3 days, sometimes 5.

I preferred to "heal" strangers because I had seen Carlos' promiscuity, and I condoned it. I'm sure that if you asked him, I was, in his eyes, promiscuous myself, albeit tamer.

There is a saying, "Familiarity breeds contempt." Not that I'm contemptuous, but I did not feel comfortable asking God for healing as if it were just a parlor game, for someone I knew was in no odyssey to better himself.

The Bible mentioned Jesus healing someone, then letting the person go about his way. If he had any instructions, sometimes he told the person he just healed not to talk about the healing that just happened, or to go straight home, instead of going to the village.

Jesus never said, "Now that I've healed you, I want you to change your life for the better."

On the one hand, I'm not Jesus, and I'm not about to tell friends, "I'll try to do my hocus pocus on you, there are no guarantees, but I require that you change your life for the better, because I'm conflicted. Your promiscuity gets in the way of miracles."

On the other hand, the basis for our friendship was looking at other people with either lust or disdain. We hung out at the bars and clubs encouraging one another to get lucky with strangers. I had seen Carlos go home with people he just met and I was indifferent. I had always felt that asking God for temporary relief of his gout attack will not work. I knew him too much.

Add the fact that he was silently indifferent.

When I threw out my sister, he knew about it. The reason I was poor at that time, was that I did not get into a high-paying medical study, because I too had a slightly elevated uric acid level in my system, a precursor to gout. He had gout medication then. I asked if he can spare a few tablets. He blatantly said that his medication was for him alone, and that I should find a way to get some for myself.

☙

More than a decade before, I tried laying on of hands on someone with HIV/AIDS. Let's call him Peter. Peter was okay with me laying hands on him. He was already sick. I wanted feedback. I thought maybe we could discuss psychic healing to improve it or abandon it if it was all just imaginary and mentally taxing. I told him this was an experiment based on my beliefs and the fact that I had spent time with a psychic surgeon.

I thought that if his T-cells increased, then I could continue doing my laying on of hands on him.

While Peter allowed me to work my magic on him several times, I never got any feedback at all—no comments nor thanks from Peter. It made me feel uncomfortable about the situation. I blamed myself for putting Peter and I into this situation of imagined hope.

Before Peter and I became friends, Peter and Carlos were friends. I'm sure Peter and Carlos talked about me and my weird interest in psychic healing. Later on, Peter changed his attitude towards me. He treated me like I was inferior to him, and then he and I, long story short, ended up rejecting one another. It turned out that there was another person he hated the most within our group, but he bunched us up as one hated group of former friends.

⁂

I got on television, print and radio in 1996 in Chicago, for an artistic statement. I will talk about this again later.

For the point I'm driving at in this chapter, during the time when my picture and accompanying interview were in the current issue of a monthly free paper, I was one day at a bookstore with a cafe. I was relaxing, drinking coffee, having dessert and skimming through some books I brought to my table, when this person, a friend of a friend, someone I had met in the past, also happened to be there.

He came up to me and asked if I had some time to talk. I said yes.

He said he had been going to a psychologist, or was it a psychiatrist, because he was unhappy with his job as a respiratory therapist. He had wanted to pursue art instead. He said he painted watercolors. Meanwhile, there I was, he said, I get on television and print, and I seemed to be okay with what I was doing being an artist.

I told him I cannot advise him. Whatever he did or wanted for himself will have to be his own decision. His career as a respiratory therapist was more stable and financially rewarding than my being an artist. I also said I was not always happy with my art and life. I just did what I felt I wanted to do, letting the chips fall where they may.

He thanked me and went back to his table.

Through the years, as I saw him, since we had mutual friends and acquaintances and similar parties, I had always perceived his look of hate and contempt at me. It seemed to me that from that day forward, he hated baring his soul to me, only to get nothing much. I also probably served as a reminder that he probably should have become an artist.

I had always thought that if you really were an artist, or a writer, or both, you would had always found a way to do it anyway.

I had always felt sorry for him. I had put in decades of art and writing, and I may still not even have a pot to piss in, but I have kept on going. I know that when it rains, it pours. I have something to look forward to. It may be tomorrow or next week or when I turn 100. Through the years, I knew he had made money and some accomplishments from his profession, but he had continued to be unhappy living his life. Someday he'll see my success, all he will have for me is even more spite.

Sometimes I thought, if he had not painted watercolors or whatever through the years, maybe it was my public appearances that he was after. He wanted the icing without the cake.

I believe that where I am, I was placed by God. I have beliefs that I have always had that kept me going. Sometimes, belief becomes fact. They manifest in the physical world. I have strange stories that involved me and the advancement of my ambitions.

I have had hunches that I'm not the only force in charge of myself.

In 2012, I saw my name "Val" and "Zubiri" in the English version of the Book of Chronicles using the Bible Code, the equidistant letter sequencing program. It's good to be mentioned by God. These little snippets have kept me going.

My pursuits are almost impossible. I want to become a famous artist who wants to charge 7 and 8 dollar figures for his art. I want to become a famous writer. I even write scripts and musicals. I will be amiss if I didn't say I had fantasized winning an Oscar and a Tony, not just for writing, but maybe for directing as well.

For all I know, for example, when I return several times to edit my writing, I continue to see errors and the need for more edits. I could just be kidding myself. I could be delusional. I could have the Messiah complex. But I *have* shown undeniable persistence and improvements in my crafts of choice.

As you get older, and as you ascend, even just mentally, you will realize that there are some negatrons in your life that you do not need to be around with. These negatrons *will* manifest themselves. You, or they, will find a way to get out of the relationship.

As you learn more and feel like you are ascending, you will find yourself connecting with others who are supportive and into the same thing.

Like me, as I make better art, more and more galleries have started to interact with me. As I write more books, more and more people come up to praise and respect me. I look forward to new friends and new respect. It is too bad that I have to leave negatrons and disrespect behind in order to pursue a difficult but most rewarding future.

֎

Like Richard Bach's *Jonathan Livingston Seagull*, we will never be alone wherever we are or end up being, but if we want to ascend and take ourselves farther up, some people won't like it.

Chapter 24

I Am an Artist & a Writer

You must know that I am officially an artist and a writer. I'd like to deny everything else.

I am not a healer. I think what I can do is hypnosis. I might be wrong. Oops, I shouldn't say that. I cannot do psychic surgery. I am merely going to be recounting in some later chapters what a Filipino psychic surgeon told me a little less than 30 years ago. 28 years ago to be exact.

Imagine information from the '50s only being published now. This is totally antiquated. Nobody should care to read this now. If you continue to want to read this, you still have a choice to go away. Stop.

This is a spiral from here, not necessarily downward. Oops.

Whatever it is, I might change your paradigm.

Here is one consolation.

As far as my art is concerned, I am aware that I should give it no less than my 100%, maybe even more. As far as my writing is concerned, I am also aware that I should give it no less than 100%.

These two, art and writing, are different fields. I cannot just give 50% in one and 50% in the other to make an acceptable 100%. This amounts to mediocrity in both. I'm trying to succeed in both fields. I probably needed to give quadruple more efforts, just to become accepted.

You may not like my art, nor my writing, but what I can tell you right now is that I am doing my best in both, for you and for the rest of the world, for whatever they are worth.

When it comes to psychic healing, I will do my best to be honest with you. None of the information are contrived. If I say I heard it elsewhere, then I heard it elsewhere.

I have been telling people that I am confident that I can conduct a weeklong workshop on making contemporary porcelain art dolls. With this art, there were so many aspects I had to master, but there is always something new to learn and discover.

The same goes for writing memoirs. I can't say I'm an expert yet, but being someone who has written a few memoirs, amongst a sea of people who have stated that they will eventually write one, but cannot or have not, I think I can also do a writer's workshop. I still have trouble with prepositions and idioms. I like to think I have a style that reflects the fact that I grew up in two countries with a variety of languages.

I must be honest with you about this book. This book amounts to skipping stones on water. I'm playing with the surface. There's something lurking deep below it. Hmm. Maybe, after reading everything, you might discover I can also give a weeklong seminar on the topic of psychic healing and psychic surgery.

I actually designed it this way. It's a memoir of my stranger experiences and thoughts as it led to, encountered and went past my time with the psychic surgeon.

This is not like a self-improvement book. Psychic surgery, psychic healing and faith healing are so much more taxing. It's not about changing your life so that you end up with a rich spouse and an expensive car. Jesus did miraculous healing 2000 years ago. He ended up crucified. This book is more about warning you that you might experience a milder form of crucifixion in your life.

❧

Imagine Christ in his time, when he was alive. Zoom out and imagine the population. Zoom in again and imagine a house where a writer lived. I would be that writer. You would be better off living with me in that house. Don't try to be Christ.

Maybe I could fit a better role. Imagine Pontius Pilate, who washed his hands of responsibility, yet remained a key character in the story. I would be Pontius Pilate. When you begin to experience or exhibit things you were not expecting, you might want to see yourself as Pontius Pilate as well. Maybe imagine being someone behind him.

Imagine the story of Jonah and the whale. To me, Jonah was someone who was given a mission. He knew it. God told him what it was. Jonah had faith, but he probably tested his fate. He probably procrastinated. He probably danced around the issue that was his mission. Jonah, the great procrastinator. 10 steps forward, and 9 steps back. Hesitate, procrastinate, hesitate, procrastinate.

Yet, however he delayed his mission, it still happened. I would be Jonah. I probably was asked to write this book. I did not want to. It took me close to 30 years to do it. I still did it. Imagine yourself as Jonah. Don't try to be better.

You might be thinking you can succeed building the next miraculous Tower of Babel. I don't endorse that. Hesitate and procrastinate. Think things through.

I may be writing about stories from my past, but what I am hoping to impart are my thoughts and lessons learned. You must sense the warning labels.

Imagine the Pope saying mass. Imagine everyone in the cathedral focused on him. Imagine being with the crowd. Next to you, imagine a homeless man and a book from his pocket fell out. You picked up the book to return to him. That would be this book. Unimportant and being read by an unimportant person. You wonder if he even read it. That book would be this book. I wrote this to be noticed, yet I hesitate to share it.

This is not the grail of grails. Jesus Christ never got rich when he healed people 2,000 years ago. The psychic surgeon never got rich doing this 30 years ago. Good luck if that is what you are after.

This is why I tell people, without even telling them that I just *might* be able to heal, that I am only an artist and a writer.

Chapter 25

Getting a Wish to Come True

While in college, I bought books on self-improvement, self-hypnosis and what might be called the occult.

A few days ago, I was watching a YouTube video and the guy defined "occult" as something that is just more unknown at the present. I had always thought that the occult is something so mysterious that it will never be proven right nor wrong.

More than 30 years ago, my definition of the word "occult" was "self-improvement through more unconventional beliefs and methods of self-hypnosis and autosuggestion."

⁂

Around that time, I bought a book that was classified under occult and metaphysics, and it had exercises for the mind.

In one procedure, you get seated in a darkened room, with palms up. You imagine the presence of the "Great Cosmic Mind." Once you are in its presence, make a request. Wait for some sort of an "answer," that the request had just been granted and it will soon come true. It could be hearing an imaginary voice, saying "It is done."

The book has not been reprinted since the '80s, but the author had passed away and there are newer, more popular terms in use now. The "law of attraction" is a new phrase.

⁂

So here was what I did, based on that and a few books from the '80s. I was merely testing the efficacy of this exercise. This was already around the time that I was already familiar with the psychic surgeon and I was almost finished writing my paper.

I imagined the Great Cosmic Mind, melding with my own subconscious mind.

I pretty much said, if all this were true, I want a trip to the United States in a month's time.

I was in a darkened room.

I concentrated, eyes closed, seated straight on a chair, with my palms facing up, rested on my knees. I sent my request out. I concentrated, believing that the Great Cosmic Mind was doing its work. I was waiting for an imaginary audible "It is done" message.

Sure enough, I heard that phrase in my mind after about three minutes of waiting.

Within a few days, Uncle Nimitz, a brother of Mama, called and asked to talk to me. He asked about school, I said it was okay, I was graduating in a few months and as soon as I submitted a term paper, I will be free.

Guess what, out of the blue, he asked me if I wanted to come visit him in the U.S.! I said yes, that would be great.

He sent me some money for the plane fare, which I bought in Manila. We had a distant relative who worked as a travel agent and we always used her for our trips.

In a month's time, I was on the plane, headed for Chicago.

☙

Here's something else that I did. 30 years ago, I asked for fame and fortune. Same thing, I did hear in my mind that the request was going to happen.

It has not happened yet.

Chapter 26

Marketing Study Points of View

Downtown Chicago has a good number of companies which do both marketing studies and mock juries.

I observed that I usually tended to side with the minority vote, in both marketing studies and mock juries. Something must be wrong with me because I saw things differently than most.

The marketing studies were sponsored by commercial companies, usually with products to promote to the public. One time, I did one where this liquor company wanted our opinions on which magazine ad designs might work best for the public. The ones I chose, which I thought were the best, were the ones most people thought were the most inferior.

Then again, I was thinking those ad agencies were up to something more subliminal, and maybe I was picking up on what they wanted. Sometimes, what people choose up front may be the weakest, most forgettable options in the selection. That's just a theory on my part.

Or maybe it's the other way around. Whatever it is, I usually ended up siding with the minority.

The mock juries were usually sponsored by opposing law firms. The law firms presented their sides and evidence to us members of the mock jury for a day, sometimes two days, to see how far they were with their arguments and to see which side might win based on the mock jury's perceptions and conclusions. This was an attempt on both sides to save time and money, because an actual lawsuit might cost their clients so much more in fees and time than an out of court settlement.

Here is a warning label for you.

These marketing studies and mock juries are about normal perception. When you come home at 5 p.m. you forget about what transpired during the day or the two days.

Faith healing, psychic healing and psychic surgery—they will change perceptions 24/7. You'll bring it home with you.

It's not 9-5. It's Life/365/24/7.

Chapter 27

Papa Gets Sick

My former neighbor Terra left Chicago to work elsewhere, but whenever she passed by, she stayed with Karen, another neighbor of mine, who lived on the first floor, and then she'll buzz me to pay me a visit.

In August 2013, she buzzed me and came up to my place. I was glad to see her, because she had seen my doll art improve over the course of 2 years. After struggling with porcelain, I struggled with more challenges. I had to figure out how to make the hair, put makeup and features using china paint, make clothes, jewelry and shoes. When she buzzed me, I finally finished all the rest of these less than a week before. I had an exciting and proud show and tell. She did too.

She mentioned that she ordered 35% food grade hydrogen peroxide and it should help to improve her health. She said you only need a few drops in water to drink once in a while. She said if I wanted some, she can give me some to try. I said no thanks, I'll read on the treatment later and buy some for myself once I decide that I could also use it. We shifted to another topic.

After visiting with me, she left Karen. She drove to another state.

As I type this, it is August 31, 2013.

In April 2013, Papa and Dinna called. They said Papa had stomach pain, and they were going to the doctor.

A week after that call, they called again. Papa had a scan and they saw a marble-sized cyst in the pancreas, but there was no need to worry. They still didn't know what it was. Hopefully it would disappear, according to the doctor. Papa was given pain medication.

This month, a week after Terra came for a visit, Papa and Dinna called again. They said the cyst from April had grown, and based on the elevated enzymes from his blood test, it was cancer. No one knew yet except myself, them, Mama and Kuya Jing.

My sister Amelia had not known yet. They wanted her to fly all the way from the island of Bohol so that they can give her the news, as she sat front and center, like some episode of This is Your Life.

I thought that was stupid. Amelia had to fly all the way to Manila to get the news?

We talked for a while. I thought that cancer can be cured, based on what I had read. I told them I had started reading about cancer when Aunt Li was still alive. I promised to read some more.

They said the doctors had decided not to operate on Papa, nor have him undergo chemotherapy nor radiation therapy. He might not survive any of these.

I told them, in a way, that was good news, because we can try alternative therapies that should be milder on him. I was optimistic and saw cancer as an irritation, a temporary disruption.

Kuya Jing called me that same day. We both agreed it was stupid for Amel to fly. It was Dinna's idea.

They eventually let Amel know over the phone.

For the next few days, I went online. I got to YouTube, where there were documentaries and views about cancer and its alternative treatments. I discovered two cheap ways to combat it. The testimonials by people who had it and were now cancer-free were convincing.

One treatment was to drink a glass of distilled water mixed with a few drops of 35% food grade hydrogen peroxide, taken three times a day, everyday until the cancer disappeared. One video by a doctor showed two patients who got cured from the hydrogen peroxide treatment. He explained that the treatment was cheap and cannot be patented, which was why doctors and drug companies will never endorse it.

Another treatment was to drink a glass of distilled water mixed with 2 teaspoons of baking soda and 2 teaspoons of maple syrup. The baking soda will supposedly kill the cancer cells because it has a basic or alkali nature. The way to get the baking soda to the cancer cells was by mixing it with the maple syrup, since cancer cells liked sugar.

Whether these "cures" were true or not, once again, Papa was dying and the doctors had given up on him.

The idea was to make the body alkali. According to some websites and YouTube videos, cancer develops in an acidic body which is usually a result of bad diet and stress.

Through the years, my family called me to say hello. Sometimes, they told me that they were just so busy that their dinner was fried chicken from the food chains.

On a call a week before the cancer diagnosis, Papa had mentioned that his "good health" was from taking fish oil capsules, cod liver oil emulsion, vitamin E and multivitamins.

I told him he probably overdosed on the fish oil. He probably should stop those fish supplements and vitamin E, which was also oil-based.

What was weird was that Terra made me aware of hydrogen peroxide a week before they called me about Papa's cancer.

I took Terra's visit as a sign from God.

෴

I reminded them about my encounter with the psychic surgeon. Maybe Papa can go to one.

෴

When Aunt Li came back to the Philippines, I told them about psychic healers, with a little more detail and urgency, telling them to find one because I believed that Aunt Li can still get better.

However, I had a feeling that all of them really just wanted her to pass away. Aunt Li lived with Papa's brother and sister-in-law who were both doctors and Christian preachers. It occurred to me that they probably saw Aunt Li's deterioration as her great opportunity to go to heaven.

I asked Kuya Jing to research on psychic healers for Aunt Li. I asked Papa to encourage Kuya Jing to do so. None of them bothered, not that I blamed them. Aunt Li was with the doctor preachers.

She got weaker and deteriorated some more.

This was when I emailed her about my discovery of the graviola of Brazil, also called "guanabana" in the U.S., which turned out to be the local Philippine "guyabano," which we also called "soursop." The guyabano is a sweet-sour fruit with white pulp, readily found in the Philippines. All they needed to do was find a grower so they can make tea from the leaves.

No one bothered. Or did they?

Now, my dad had cancer. He said that when I told him about the guyabano leaf tea regimen, he did buy a plant and it was now about 9 feet tall. He started making tea for himself. I asked him how he prepared them. He said he boiled them until the water got dark. I told him he boiled too much of it, and that was a lot of chlorophyll which might be bad. I told him to just make enough from 2 or 3 small leaves at a time, and drink the water while it was still just a light green hue, much like the color of green tea.

I was guessing, but I tried to be authoritative about it. I pretended I knew what I was talking about.

Mama had stomach problems and got hospitalized decades ago when she drank what Filipino herbalists called "7-7," a boiled concoction from 7 leaves which were sold by herbalists, which was supposed to be cleansing and slimming. She drank copious amounts of the dark liquid and ended up in the hospital.

Aunt Li was very sick anyway. We all accepted that she was dying. Papa never told me he bothered to buy a guyabano plant. When? Why didn't he bother to inform me? Bad thoughts came to mind, but now he's sick. I thought I will argue with him as soon as he got himself clear of cancer.

Papa called a few times after his cancer news. I had been telling them to get the 35% food grade hydrogen peroxide mixed with distilled water. They were able to buy the distilled water, but the only hydrogen peroxide they found at the drugstores were the 3% topical solution for wounds and the one used for bleaching hair. I told them to keep looking for it, but if they really can't find it, they can start with the baking soda treatment, but with instructions to call me as soon as they have the ingredients in front of them.

☙

I got a phone call again.

Papa was very cheerful, like he had good news to tell me.

"Thanks for the tip about the baking soda. I saw the doctor and he said it would work," he said.

I asked, "Good. So you took it?"

"Only once," he said. "But my blood pressure shot up. The doctor said it would work on me if I were healthy. But since my blood pressure went up, we're stopping it."

I got mad. I asked, "When did this happen?"

"Oh, two days ago."

I got mad. "Didn't I tell you to call me the moment you were going to do all this?"

"We were busy. We were doing errands."

"Didn't I tell you that you will need to rest and lie down because the treatment will have side effects?"

"Well how many days do you want me to do nothing but lie down?"

"What have you been up to?"

"We're working on the papers for our properties."

"Papa, you had your entire life, so many years to do whatever it is you need to do with those legalities. Now you're sick and dying, you need to lie down and try to get better!" I shouted.

"What do you want me to do? Die sooner from a heart attack? I told you my blood pressure shot up when I did what you told me to do!" he answered back.

"Did you watch those videos from YouTube I sent you?"

"No."

"Not one of them?"

"No, what do you want me to do? Spend my entire day watching videos?"

"If you watched them, you would be motivated at the very least!"

☙

All this time, I had been working on a new batch of dolls. I saw my landlord, Richard, downstairs, so when I said hello, I told him I wanted to show him my art.

As I was showing Richard my art, I told him my dad had pancreatic cancer. He praised my work. He also told me not to worry about my rent yet, just worry about my dad.

After seeing Richard, I decided to see my first floor neighbor Karen to show her my work, since I had them with me already. She let me into her apartment. I showed her my work, she praised it as usual. Through the years, she and Terra had seen the progression of my work. It was the first time she saw them finished. Karen seemed a little high on something. Sure enough, she lit a pipe. Medical marijuana.

I told her my dad had pancreatic cancer.

What came out of her was another coincidence. She said "Oh, by the way, in the '70s, I went to the burbs and this psychic surgeon from the Philippines took out a golf-sized tissue out of my stomach, after which I felt better."

I was a little taken aback. She never mentioned this in the past. I told her I have my own stories about psychic surgery. I told her that my English term paper in college was about it.

We talked some more until someone from the sidewalk shouted her name. She looked out and told me she needed to let the lady in. I said goodbye, and she walked out with me so she can let the lady in.

As we exchanged a few last sentences, she said, "Oh, my next door neighbor Jules has cancer too, but he's stage 3 or even worse. He's going to the vet to get treated."

"Vet? Like the veterinarian?" I laughed.

"No, silly. The VA. Veterans Hospital. He fought in the Gulf War," she said, laughing.

"Who you talking about? Do I know him?" I asked.

"Yeah! That guy who always sits at the steps."

"Dink?"

"Yes, him! His name is Jules. What do you mean 'Dink'? His nickname's 'Dank'!"

There was this neighbor I met last year at the laundry room. He and I were doing our laundry, and he called himself "Dink." I thought I heard "Dink."

Karen just last month mentioned him and explained that "Dank" meant something related to incredibly good, awesome, high-quality marijuana. I Googled the word, and it was spelled "Dank." In my mind, "Dink" stuck.

As Karen explained the nickname, it was obvious she didn't like it. That must have been why she referred to him as "Jules," his real name.

I had always seen him outside our building, socializing with people on the streets. I think I finally understood his name. He probably gave himself that nickname so people knew whom to call for some high-quality dank. Well, I had no plans to buy any weed, I didn't really care about his connection to weed.

I saw some documentaries about cannabis or marijuana. They said it stopped cancer and, being that it is a naturally-occurring hallucinogen it might had helped the caveman evolve into modern, thinking human beings.

I thought he was an okay guy, but I heard from one of my building managers that some UPS or FedEx deliveries were received by someone from my building, but those packages never reached my neighbors. The building managers suspected that Dank, the only one who was always in front of the building, stole them.

So now, Karen told me that Dank had just been diagnosed with late stage cancer, and it had spread out to different parts of his body. Because I had been researching on alternative treatments for cancer, I had thought about giving him some suggestions. She said that Dank was going to get either chemotherapy, radiation therapy or both, from the VA.

My perception of Dank flip-flopped. I first met him in the laundry room in the basement last year. I liked him. Then I heard about the lost packages and learned what his nickname meant. I liked him less. Then I heard about his cancer and Gulf War service. My perception of him flipped again.

Should I pray for his health and healing or leave him alone?

*

All of these recent events in August 2013 seemed to be a sign for me to write and finish this book on healing soon.

Chapter 28

Kansas City Danny

In 2012, I was in Kansas City volunteering for a medical study as, what else, a medical study subject. A laboratory rat. A lab rat. The study I was in used 16 men. We stayed in the medical facility for about three weeks. The place was filled to capacity, with about a total of 100 subjects, both male and female. There were several studies of different drugs happening at the same time, with different durations. As a group left, another came in.

I was obviously Asian. There was another Asian-looking man, but I suspected he was mixed. I suspected he was Korean and white. I stayed away from him.

Everyday, I saw him in the hallway, uncaring of whoever was there. With his eyes closed, he was frozen in a pose, as if he was doing some sort of an Asian type of meditation. He looked awkward. He did not care who saw him that way.

My room had 14 electric hospital beds for the people in my study. The last two guys stayed in a different room, with other people in a different study. We roommates all eventually got used to one another, since we didn't have a choice. The supervisors tried to squeeze two more beds in, but it was impossible.

When the subject of the weird Asian guy outside came up in my room, I also put my two cents in. Like my roommates, I too thought he was weird. Someone asked me if I had talked to him, and I said no.

I eventually learned that the Asian guy's study was ending in a few days. I finally decided to approach him.

"What were those poses for?" I asked.

"I was meditating," he answered.

"Oh? What else do you do?" I asked.

"Martial arts. I teach martial arts."

"I'm an artist and a writer. Wanna see my work?" I asked.

"Sure."

I went to my room to get my laptop. I had been photoediting the latest pictures of my dollwork to post on my doll blog, so I showed him my pictures. Then I told him that my latest book, ***Dollman the Musical, A Memoir of an Artist as a Dollmaker*** was available online. I went online and showed him the listing on Barnes and Noble.com.

He pointed to my other books. "Are those yours as well?"

I answered, "Yeah, from years back. This one is a collection of nude drawings and paintings from 1995 to 1996, and the other one is about psychic surgery, but the one on psychic surgery is a collection of chapters from another book, ***Memoir of an Artist as a Masseur***, which I pulled out. I need to reedit the masseur book. I started thinking it was too long."

"You wrote ***Healing Lessons from a Psychic Surgeon?***" he asked.

"Yes, but the book contains chapters from the bigger masseur memoir book, so I cheated. While I took out the big masseur memoir, I made sure I had the psychic surgery book out." I explained.

"I know what you did. I may have read your book. I ordered it a while back."

"You did? Wow! You're one of the few who bought it?" I laughed.

"Yeah," he said.

"Why?" I asked.

"I wanted to learn about psychic surgery, and your book was the only one available who teaches it."

"Oh wow! Did you like it?" I asked, flustered.

"Yeah, it was good."

"We should have met earlier! If you had questions, I could have answered it!"

☙

In my mind, I was telling myself that I contributed to Danny's weirdness. I saw Danny as a sign for me to look back and redo my book, ***Healing Lessons from a Psychic Surgeon.***

This book is my redo, thanks to Danny.

CHAPTER 29

PAPA GETS SICK 2

As I said earlier, expect opposition from known and unknown forces. I'm not talking about angels and demons. I'm talking about immediate family members.

When my family called to tell me that Papa had pancreatic cancer, not only did I tell Dinna that I was going to research on it, I also told her, over the phone, how to pray for Papa's healing, based on the instructions of the psychic surgeon.

Dinna agreed with the "methodology." She said she can do it. I didn't trust her. She promised to call me everyday so I can join them when they prayed. They did call me, but only once.

Dinna wanted a précis of my composition. A few lines of summarized text in email form, from my cellphone to hers, to save a life.

There was no need to prep her that it might not just be life-saving, it might also be life-changing.

She simply said in passing that whatever I text her, she will do with such easy nonchalant reassurance. When I got that from her, a vision of myself successfully teaching a horse psychic surgery and psychic healing, that thing which changed the course of my life, came to my mind.

I hate to say this, but they reassured me in April that whatever tiny, marble-sized scarring Papa had in his pancreas was "probably" nothing I should worry about. Then in August they told me he definitely had cancer and that marble got bigger. Those were four lost months of alternative therapy.

They had baking soda in the cupboard. They were able to get distilled water at the grocery. The baking soda regimen supposedly had astonishing results after 2 or 3 days of use. They were only able to do it once. They never bothered to call me back to update me.

I wondered what if they did this four months ago? They reassured me that whatever Papa had was nothing to worry about.

Based on what I understood from the videos, about the baking soda treatment, the baking soda can burst the outer layer of cancer with just the first treatment. I had the idea that as soon as they started the treatment, they had to keep doing it for the few days to probably a week. If they burst the cancer, then cancer cells would be floating about in his system within the two days that they did not bother to call me.

If I had cancer, I would do what was necessary and lie down, expecting to feel sick before I begin to recover. Papa did not have a headache. He had cancer. They wanted their cake and eat it too.

I then reminded them, especially Kuya Jing to keep looking for the 35% food grade hydrogen peroxide. He finally found a source—three weeks later. He was able to buy it the following day.

In retrospect, I probably made a mistake as well. I should have encouraged them to look for hydrogen peroxide before suggesting the baking soda. The problem I had with them was that they did not want to communicate with me as promptly as I asked them to do so.

I cannot really fault myself. Papa was getting old. They said he can spend days in front of his computer, supposedly doing stuff about the properties he inherited, but throughout so many years, nothing much progressed.

He also spent time online, but to watch a few minutes of videos to fight his cancer was out of the question.

We had an online phone subscription, and for years, we talked for hours, distance didn't matter, but he never showed nor told me any worries about his marble sized "scarring" and none of them even volunteered what the doctors thought it was except that they needed to wait and see if the thing disappeared from the scans.

When we talked about food, Papa enumerated the bad food they ate, such as eating a bucket of fried chicken, because they were too busy, or how much he loved sardines, despite the fact that all of them had high uric acid.

All this time, from the time I had started to endorse the baking soda and the hydrogen peroxide regimens, I was also telling them to look for litmus paper strips. It will be in a box that has a color chart, either on the box or inside the box, printed on the insert.

According to internet articles and YouTube videos, in order to find out if a person had an acidic system, they should test both the morning saliva and the morning urine. A person with cancer will show an acidic system, and the litmus paper will show this. Cancer thrives in an acidic body.

Papa's system needed to turn alkali. If he followed either the baking soda or the hydrogen peroxide regimen for a few days to two weeks, the litmus paper strips should, hopefully, show a gradual change in color, from acidic to alkali, and as the color changes, we will have an idea of how to regulate the regimen.

Kuya Jing and I went to pre-medicine. Both of us have a Bachelors Degree in Biology. We had at least three chemistry classes coupled with laboratory time. We knew what litmus paper looked like. We encountered hydrogen peroxide. They existed in Manila. Why they cannot find litmus paper and hydrogen peroxide for the longest time was beyond me.

Mama was a pharmacy student before she shifted to another course. She also had knowledge of chemicals.

I went online again, and discovered that litmus paper was also more commonly called "pH strips." I told them to look for "pH strips," not litmus paper. The were never able to find any source for pH paper.

I had explained to them that they only needed a few drops of hydrogen peroxide in a glass of distilled water. I had explained to them that distilled water was to be used, because the few drops of hydrogen peroxide would immediately react with impurities in anything other than distilled water. If tap water had any impurities, the hydrogen peroxide would react with it first, possibly dissipating its efficacy before Papa even ingested it.

The goal was to get the hydrogen peroxide into Papa's system, not to cleanse the medium it was in.

And so time came when Kuya Jing finally found 35% food grade hydrogen peroxide.

He put 6 drops of hydrogen peroxide in some great tasting aloe vera juice. In my mind, putting 6 drops of hydrogen peroxide in muddy, murky water from the canal outside the house would have been just as effective.

At least he immediately updated me about it. I emailed him back. I told him that they were supposed to use distilled water with the hydrogen peroxide. Once again I reminded them to call me the moment they were going to do it. He relayed the message to Dinna and Papa because he just got home, 2 hours away from Manila. They resolved to do it the next day.

That next day did not happen. Kuya Jing texted me again. They were bringing Papa to the hospital, because Dinna, Papa and Mama prayed the rosary. Papa knelt, and then squatted like a healthy American Indian. His left leg fell asleep. It had been two hours since and his leg just would not regain its sensation.

According to the YouTube testimonials, some cancers went away in just a day or two of hydrogen peroxide treatments, just like the claims from the baking soda regimen. The videos seemed incredible, but that was what the people in the videos were saying. Kuya Jing had eventually seen some of the videos. Dinna and Papa had separate computers—they never yet bothered to watch any 7 to 10 minute YouTube videos, even after a month of dealing with Papa's pancreatic cancer.

If I lived with them, this chapter would be longer. Maybe shorter. Who knows.

My gut instinct told me that Papa will never heed my suggested methods.

I'm sharing this frustration in this book, because, as I had been saying, there will be opposition to all this on many levels. While the rare paranormal is involved in my rhetoric here, my barriers included the daily normal.

☙

The moment you acknowledge that you would be on a mission for this great invisible force that is God, and you get interested in psychic healing, you will feel competition between good and evil. It may or may not scare you, but it will become more and more tangible in your entire existence, even if you can't do it yet.

You will come to realize that those closest to you will be the ones who will want to hear you the least.

My brother and I had been texting. He had the same argument. Papa, Mama and Dinna will do what they can based on their own interpretations. Papa was hospitalized for his sleeping left leg. His leg got better, but according to Kuya Jing, he seemed to like the simple thought of just being with doctors, who all had told him there was nothing more they can do to cure him. I told him, let's just wait for him to get worse and desperate, and at that moment, see if he decides to heed us.

I got the feeling that Papa wanted a cure for his pancreatic cancer as long as it had no side effects. He wanted his cake and eat it too.

Papa wanted us to become doctors. We refused. We can't possibly be smart like the doctors.

☙

Here I was, writing about my beloved Papa, and I was letting him go.

I got the feeling that he just wanted to prove my suggestions wrong, and he was willing to die to prove himself right. He made some comments about me not being there to help out anyway.

Dinna had always been a religious person. She wanted to become a nun in the past. I cannot blame her if she thought the psychic surgeon's methods were off. It can be easy for her to say that Papa's condition was God's will. Her life decision was to stay with Papa and Mama to take care of them. I was sure she did what she can. On a daily basis, maybe she had tired of it. My own contention has been, that we had relatives who lived past 95. Mama's own dad lived to be 100. In my mind, I saw my parents as they were 50 years ago. Dinna saw them daily. Papa had gotten old through the years. I was just not having it.

This book on healing that I am writing, close to 30 years after my encounter with a Filipino psychic surgeon became my therapy in dealing with Papa's illness. There had been strange coincidences that seemed to have come from the unknown, God or otherwise, which seemed to tell me that it was time to write this. Maybe I found Papa's condition as an excuse to add the needed dimension to write this book. I was actually planning to write something else.

☙

I decided that if I can't help my dad, maybe this book is for a bigger audience. You, the stranger who does not know me from beans who will find it valuable to listen to me and heed everything I have to say: the fine prints, the warning labels, the riddles and the how-tos. Maybe, if I can't do the psychic healing myself, there will be at least one person out there who will accept the challenge. Maybe my mission was to write this. Maybe that's all I was supposed to do. Someone else will continue whatever the next stage will be. It could be you.

My sin, my crime, was that I became serious about this because Papa was dying.

☙

People, in general, want their cake and eat it too. I'm that way as well. There are those who chase miracles all over the place, even going out of their countries to do so, when all the while the faith should come from within them.

I like to think I'm a good person. I have my standards. I cannot expect people to fall within my standards. Some people think I'm not a good person. They think they are better. I cannot fall within their own standards.

You will encounter people who are sick, who will want instant cures, but without their guarantees that they in exchange will begin to watch their ways, physical or otherwise, that they will guarantee healthier living, or live a less promiscuous life, or that they will stop stealing other people's deliveries.

We all had encountered many people who never thanked us for favors. Their numbers will grow. It's insulting and belittling if we allow them to eat into our being. We should respond to and interact with God, more than we allow ourselves to be affected by the neutral non-action, passive disinterest and negative actions of other fellow human beings.

☙

Here, finally, is a fine print. Psychic healing is faith healing.

According to the psychic surgeon, his power came from God. Only his faith mattered. The people who approached him, and who will approach you and I, they need not change.

Psychic healing is a draining existence, even as you claim that it is God's energy you are using, it will drain you.

If you were the chosen one, will you be able to change the world? Was Christ able to change the world? He still got crucified. As you move forward with this, be aware of your limits and the limits of others, especially those around you.

Riddles. Maybe I'm being melodramatic. You will discover that you will need to do more than you do now to effect psychic power. If you just want to be normal, there's no need to proceed. We probably should just do what we can. Maybe that's all that God has been asking us.

Chapter 30

Our Doomsday Generation

This current generation seems to be a strange one.

People, including myself, anticipated that some computer systems will fail at the turn of the millennium. Nothing happened, but I heeded warnings.

I bought a book with a checklist of things to do to prepare for disaster. I disinfected and cleaned my bathtub, and filled it with water, just in case the water supply stopped working.

When 9/11 happened, I saw silent panic. I lived in downtown Chicago. On that day, and for the next few days, no one walked on the downtown sidewalks unless they had to. No one even dared to ride a bike to exercise or pass the time. I did not see anyone running or jogging. There were almost no cars on the streets. There were less taxicabs around, probably because a lot of the non-white drivers with accents feared retaliation. It looked as if downtown was a ghost town for a few days.

For weeks, tourism and conventions froze.

I realized the importance of food and how scarce it can become in a day's notice. My apartment complex consisted of twin buildings that had a little more than 40 floors each. We had one single White Hen Pantry on the first floor. The food, including the junk food, were all gone by the night of the day after, on the 12th. Even the expensive pints of ice cream were gone.

We also had a good number of economic crashes. There was the dot-com bubble in 2000, the real estate bubble that happened at different times in almost all countries, and the downturn of the economy in 2008.

There was the end of the Mayan calendar which we thought

was the end of the world. There had been more frequent UFO sightings. There's global warming. Global ice age. There were the tsunamis that killed thousands of people. Hurricanes and typhoons that killed so much more than the usual number.

Where I live now, there is a Baptist church that helps the poor and the homeless. They open their doors at night to let the homeless sleep. They have days when they distribute food. I'm not racist, but the lines that used to form leading to the church, for whatever it was they were doing for the moment, the lines used to have only blacks and some Hispanics. In 2008, I saw a well-dressed white person in line. Nowadays, I see all different races lined up. I see old Asian ladies lining up for groceries.

In speedreading class in the late '80s, I read Hal Lindsey's book, *The Late Great Planet Earth*. It just came out as a paperback. It talked about the end of the world. Hal Lindsey is still alive. He continues to be a Christian preacher. The book became a bestseller. It foretold of Communist China invading the rest of the world.

※

Here is an observation that might prove that America is not always on the forefront. There have been some things America allowed itself to miss.

When filesharing became popular, about 15 years ago, the world began sharing files. Granted that copyrights were infringed upon, the U.S. started going after the people they can easily make examples of—its own Americans. The rest of the world continued to share files.

What was emphasized was the sharing of entertainment files—music and movies. What was not fully publicized were the sharing of software and educational books—things people can acquire skills from.

Fifteen years later, the 15-year-old filesharing kids are now 30 years old. What used to be U.S.-based programming jobs now seem to have been forked out to other countries. It seems to me that those kids elsewhere who were able to download software and instructionals through the years are the ones getting the jobs now.

Winter Olympics at Socchi, in Russia. There were television news features that showed that as soon as they arrived in Russia and used wi-fi to access the internet, their laptops immediately got hacked into. That's some great skill right there. Bad thing to do, but great skill.

I learned PHP, a programming language designed for the internet, and its matching database program, MySQL. I still can't hack a computer. Looking at the requirements for programming and internet jobs on Craigslist, I need more than PHP and MySQL to get a job. I discovered PHP in 1998, when I just started living downtown, doing massage to get my first memoir, about an artist being a masseur off and running. I still learned PHP and MySQL.

There were only 3 books on PHP when I started visiting Borders Bookstore for computer books on making websites, programming and computer graphics. If I had a question, since Borders was nearby, I hung out by the computer books and waited for people to take a book related to my question off the shelf.

Now, I can program using PHP and MySQL, almost with my eyes closed. I can be fast, but I don't think it's enough.

୫୨

Sensing when someone needed intervention.

I still hung out with some friends even after learning that my dad got cancer. I needed to cheer up. I also needed to forget the worry, depression and desperation I was experiencing because of their lack of communication with me.

Once, I went to a bar. I got drunk. I had been working on my art dolls and whenever the kiln was on, I opened my laptop to write.

On that night, I didn't mind a break. My friend George invited me for a drink.

I was at the stage in the dollwork when I had to use the kiln everyday. I painted the doll faces in stages. China paint is actually made of powdered glass. Each stage or layer in painting required that the paint be fused to the porcelain using the kiln. My typical day for the past few days had been 6 to 8 hours of china painting, followed by the kiln's 8 hours of heating up and another 6 hours of cooling down. While the kiln was on, I continued to write this book.

I was done with the draft of this book, so I went out. Connecting with the rest of the world through a drink or two once in a while is good. A change in scenery can remind me of some topic or story to add in the book. Whenever I wrote, I made sure I was sensitive to the videos I watched, or the subjects my friends and I talked about. I believed that the Great Cosmic Mind intentionally told me what to write about next.

Sitting next to me at the bar was a guy, with whom I decided to talk to. He was a little shy and the way he conducted himself gave me the idea that he was not mentally well.

This guy and I talked. He said he was depressed. He also said he behaved strangely sometimes, so I had to give him space for that.

I told him I'll make him feel better. I did my hocus pocus visualization technique on him.

He said he felt better.

I told him I was writing a book on psychic healing. When you say you're writing a book, with confidence, it gives you an air of leadership and supremacy. I realized he needed more than what I can give him. He needed psychiatric help. However, I was the one available that night that can boss him around, maybe nudge him to a better disposition.

He asked for more of my homemade visualization hocus pocus. Well, what I really did was casually touch him on his arms for just a few seconds and touch him on the head for about five seconds and no more.

Then I gave him a nice massage on his shoulder and did some visualization, but I didn't tell him this.

He actually thanked me some more. No miracle here can be proven. It's all just normal mental and emotional connection.

He also said he might never see me again, but what I was able to give him, he appreciated.

Within an hour's worth of drinks, he mentioned something crucial, in just a few sentences. When he was 13 or 15 years old, I cannot remember, I was already tipsy, his mom asked him to hand her the gun they had at home. He ran to get the gun and gave the gun to her. In front of him, his mom shot herself in the head. He said that was why he was screwed up.

I told him, "Feel better tomorrow. I'm screwed up myself, because I was molested when I was a child, but I'm okay now. You should be okay now."

Here again was a sign. I had to add him to this book. People need help one way or another.

In my mind, as I was trying to make sense of my surroundings, walking around with people walking a little more aimlessly and directionlessly than myself, I saw this man, he was part of this doomsday generation crowd.

※

In 2008, I discovered Coast to Coast AM, a nightly radio show that started around midnight, that talked about UFOs, ghosts, angels and demons and other paranormal subjects. Around 2011 or 2012, the station that delivered it in Chicago decided to discontinue it, but I discovered that some fans uploaded the show on YouTube. I still got my Coast to Coast fix on a regular basis, although it was not the live show that I was listening to anymore. The live show was more fun; maybe a Chicago radio station will bring it back.

I remember a caller asking why the show had not had the doomsday authors like Hal Lindsey on, because these earlier authors from the '70s and '80s also tackled predictions, the apocalypse, Armageddon and the end of the world. The host George Noory explained that those old authors were later proven to be wrong in their prophetic messages.

As I wrote about psychic healing and psychic surgery, I remembered Hal Lindsey. I asked myself, when will a book about psychic healing and psychic surgery be timely enough and when will it become obsolete?

Now will be a good time to release this book. In the past, a lot more people would have objected.

Had I released a book on psychic surgery and psychic healing, seemingly disguised as a memoir 30 years ago, or a memoir with mention of psychic surgery and psychic healing 30 years ago, I don't think it would had been as impactful as now.

Nowadays, people entertain the unknown. I think we now open our minds not necessarily to new ideas, but to more ideas, both old and new.

Here is an observation that I mentioned in my term paper close to 30 years ago. What I had noticed about psychic healing or faith healing in the Philippines, it existed for people who were poor and cannot afford to go to a western-trained doctor. It was a byproduct of their bad economic situation.

The Philippines continues to be poor. I am sure psychic healers and psychic surgeons are still there in abundance. When I wrote about them, 28 years ago, I said that one book mentioned that there were about 150 psychic surgeons in the country. Maybe there are more now than ever.

The world right now is in a bad economic situation.

I believe that people in America and elsewhere will entertain this, not because they have seen ghosts and UFOs, nor because they entertain the possibility of the existence of multiple dimensions. It is because more people are simply economically poor now, they cannot afford long days in hospitals and expensive medicines. It will be a while before they admit that I might be correct. Entertaining the unknown would suffice as an excuse for this interest.

At the time of this, our Doomsday Generation, there must be need for this book.

Chapter 31

Repeating Numbers

I discovered Coast to Coast around 2008. It was still broadcast in Chicago, but sometimes the signal got jammed for some reason, that I searched for other stations that had it. My radio picked up weak signals from two other big cities, both from out of state.

Strange, but Coast to Coast is online, so I have continued to listen to it, and people on occasion still complained about jamming or weak radio signals.

Coast to Coast talked about the paranormal. UFOs, ghosts, crop circles, alien abduction, and many other weird topics.

In 2008, I did not listen every night, because the program started at midnight, and ended at 4 a.m., but there was a night I caught where this caller said he kept seeing repeating numbers.

On his watch and clocks: 11:11, 12:12, 10:10. Or he looked elsewhere and he saw number patterns.

The host, George Noory, said that it must had been the caller's imagination. He had never heard of such a phenomenon. And on to the next caller.

※

What was funny was that I also saw patterns in numbers, not just repeating ones. I didn't think there was anything strange about it. It became a mind game that cheered me up at various moments of the day. I'm mentioning this here, because the caller then was serious about his observation and the host George Noory hung up too fast and switched to the next caller. I thought this could be important to numerologists. Maybe in a future show, a numerologist would tell the listeners what seeing number patterns meant.

One time, I was at KFC. I ordered something cheap, but I gave the cashier a hundred dollars.

She asked, "Do you have plans to buy a lottery ticket?"

"Why?" I asked back.

"Because here's your change. It's $97.97," she said, smiling, as she gave me my money back.

Obviously there were two of us then who noticed the repeating numbers.

※

The medical facilities I had been to all had atomic clocks. The red LED clocks were all over the place, all calibrated so that they displayed the same exact time, right down to the second. They were all set on a 24-hour cycle.

Once in a while I looked up, and saw, for example, 14:14:14, or 14:15:16. Well, 14:28:42 would be a little difficult to figure out, I don't think I would spot the pattern but 05:10:15 would be easy to notice, although to see that would mean I'm already awake and alert at 5:10 a.m. 10:20:30 or 12:23:34 might be more manageable being that they are late morning and noontime hours.

It was quite obvious that over a 24-hour period, a lot of patterns could be noticed. It was just fun to figure them out. Of course, most of the time that I looked up, there were no patterns to be noticed.

It turned out that other people noticed repeating numbers too. Where those clocks were, it was not just myself who noticed the patterns. We had fun glancing up randomly at the clocks, even as we were busy doing other things, like reading or using our laptops. A few seconds before a pattern, we alerted the rest in the room to look at the clock.

※

The thing about seeing repeating numbers, was that if you get hooked on doing it, you'll see a lot more patterns.

I for one liked doing it, because it cheered me up. Then I usually said to myself, "Oh, an invisible force just alerted me."

CHAPTER 32

SINFUL ACTS OF KINDNESS

It seemed to me that we in this generation, including both gay and straight people, with the internet and many technological devices, that we are connecting for the fun, but wrong, reasons.

I want to write another memoir.

I want to call it "Sinful Acts of Kindness."

It will be like "Random Acts of Kindness," except that it will be filled with stories of people who thought connection included random acts of sex and drugs. It will be replete with sex and promiscuity. There will be incidents of drug use.

One time I asked someone, "What's with all these people? They are rich, they get depressed, they drink and they do drugs. I get depressed but I don't drink nor do drugs."

"That's because you're poor, Val," he said. "If you wanna do drugs, you gotta have money. You can't even afford cigarettes."

❧

There is a saint, Saint Augustine, who, in a nutshell, converted to Catholicism around the age of 33. Before that, he did a lot of unacceptable things. Supposedly, his life was "hedonistic," however you or I might define that word. Four years later, he became a priest, and a few more years later he became a full bishop. He was 75 when he died.

What Saint Augustine did in his life, however, was write about being Christian and how wrong his life before Christianity had been. St. Augustine's writings had a huge impact on Catholicism.

I started praying for my dad, and I also started reading about the lives of saints. Some saints were able to perform miracles when they were still alive. Saint Pio, or Padre Pio when he was alive had stigmata, the nail wounds of Christ. He also levitated and bilocated.

☙

Going to Catholic churches, with all those statues, I noticed that a lot of the saints were priests, nuns and monks. If I wanted to become an effective holy person, capable of miracles, especially for Papa, then I should become a priest or a monk. Religious people live and breath prayer, connection with God, 24/7, while lay people had families to take care of and bills, rent and mortgages to pay.

This was why I was "recalibrating" my prayers and religiosity. I needed to be more religious to get positive results for my dad. I took time off in October and November to be able to go to daily mass and spend even more time at home to pray even more. I also finally decided to become more serious about the healing visualizations.

☙

The psychic surgeon told me that the most important thing he did was to give himself his interpretation of 40 days and 40 nights. He said that even Christ did it, going to the desert, and so he did it as well.

He took time off of work. He locked himself in his room. He prayed and read the Bible.

He said strange things happened to him. He said God made His presence felt. The bad side also made their presence felt.

The healer told me about sex. He was married and had kids. He went to work—he had a regular job. He said that I would have to make sacrifices, however I would interpret that, but just to let me know, he said that sex drained healing energy.

Because he did his healing on Sundays, he made sure he did not have any sexual activity for a few days prior to Sunday.

For someone like me, who was not really a healer like him,

my interpretation was that I would have to really just not even think about sex. I was willing to do this for my dad. No sex for weeks... however I would interpret that.

Once Papa called and I told him I was sacrificing sex to be able to pray better. I said I believed that I would be better at following what the psychic surgeon taught me to do, those visualization exercises. I also said that I erased all the porn in my hard drive.

I knew I shouldn't have had all those porn in the first place anyway. However much that was, it's all gone. By the time I made this decision, I did it willingly. Doing it was not a sacrifice at all.

The possible problem I think I had with God, I knew I was spiritual in the past, but I was not really going to church. I was afraid I was, only now, because of Papa, playing catch up.

I guess I will write something like "Sinful Acts of Kindness" in the future. I'm very guilty of something.

CHAPTER 33

ENVY

Papa's Lubang Island is a relatively tiny island that is part of a larger island. The larger island of Mindoro was big enough that it had been split into two provinces, Occidental and Oriental Mindoro, in 1950.

Lubang Island, and Cabra Islet, discussed in another chapter, are two tiny dots that belong to Occidental Mindoro, both located north and to the west of the huge island of Mindoro.

The Vietnamese boat people left Vietnam, in the late '70s, to escape the Vietnam War. What the Vietnamese did was leave their country in boats, setting out on a straight course perpendicular to their country's shore. Directly ahead, going east, is the Philippines. A good number ended up on Lubang Island, where they stayed for a while and got "processed," and waited to get to the other countries, including the United States. Filipinos and the news used the word "process." I thought it meant teaching them English.

In January 1974, a Japanese soldier from World War II, Lt. Hiroo Onoda, finally came out of hiding on Lubang Island to surrender. A Japanese adventurer Norio Suzuki heard about the soldier who did not believe that the war was over. He found Lt. Onoda and was able to convince Lt. Onoda to surrender. There were four people who hid initially—one surrendered in 1950, one died in 1954 after a shootout with a search party and another in 1972 after a shootout with the police. Mr. Suzuki, the adventurer, died in an avalanche in 1986 pursuing his own adventures. He was looking for the yeti.

As for the locals on the island, through the years, about 30 people died from the Japanese soldiers' guerilla activities. Lt. Onoda died in January 2014 at the age of 91, a hero in Japan, admired by the world, and forgiven but not forgotten by the people of Lubang Island. I'm just being melodramatic. Some people continue to hate him. My grandpa supposedly knew someone who was blinded by a booby trap of his.

❦

There was a ship that sailed at least once a week between Manila to Lubang Island. It must had been a lucrative business, because a lot of Lubang Islanders lived in Manila. In 2009, this ship, Catalyn B, sank on its way to Lubang, on Christmas Eve. I saw the list of missing passengers recognizing some last names.

❦

My grandparents used to fight a lot when they were alive. My grandma claimed that my grandpa was a womanizer. Grandpa laughed it off, but it may had been true.

Uncle Nick once lent his car and his driver to my grandpa, so he can get a haircut and a manicure. I went with him. I was in the car with the driver, while Grandpa was inside the barber shop. He was getting his haircut while getting a manicure from a middle-aged, plump lady manicurist.

Then the driver said, "Val, they want your attention."

Grandpa waved to me from the clear glass window of the shop. All the barbers were looking out as well. Grandpa pointed to his manicurist who was smiling at me as well. He kissed her on the cheek twice, making sure I saw it. I thought it was funny. I believed it was just a show he put on for me.

There was one thing my grandparents were proud of and did not fight about. Through the years, they had land on Lubang Island. When we siblings were kids and vacationed on the island, we rode on my grandparents' truck with their workers, back and forth between my grandparents' home in Tilik, which had their house and a huge *bodega*, or warehouse, and Pusong, where their salt beds were, 30 minutes away, where their workers raked sea salt from flat salt beds.

Grandma used to proudly stand on the truck as we drove on

the Main Road, past flat farmlands and hills. She pointed out the patches of land "we" owned. "We" kids were included, she considered us to be the future owners of what they had amassed.

※

My appreciation for Lubang Island and my deceased, fighting, but legendary grandparents continue to this day, because of a "warning" that I heard from them.

Because of what they owned and the success and accomplishments of their children, they used to tell us, once in a while, that we were to expect and get used to envy from people. It's a natural reaction. We should never count it against people.

※

There are things which can induce envy from people. Property, accomplishments, success, even drive and ambitions and goals that haven't even been achieved yet. If ever I became successful as an artist and a writer, some people will not like it. Actually, the mere fact that I continue to pursue art and writing, without even a pot to piss in, had been a source of envy from some people I had interacted with. Here comes another book I've written! Where's yours?

The same thing happens and will continue to happen with you. As you change for the better, there will be some who will envy you. There might even be some who will stop you.

Some people want you where they can see you.

What if you begin showing abilities related to psychic healing?

What that means is that you have become more religious than they. How dare you become a psychic healer. You're in the grace of God. Why not they?

The envy you might encounter might not even be from humans. Here is one reason why I had been dancing around the issue. As God makes his good presence felt, so will the others that don't like Him too much.

Don't feel too scared, however. It will feel like competing

street vendors trying to get your attention to buy the same thing everyone else is selling.

Welcome to the strange, mystical, mystifying adventure of your life and soul.

Chapter 34

Lessons from a Psychic Surgeon 1

I dreamt of the psychic surgeon again.

I spoke, "I remember your face, but not your name anymore."

"Do I scare you?" he asked.

"Not as much as I scare myself. I still remember your psychic healing practices. I can't do it. I was never ready to receive such a gift. I'm still not ready. I don't want the gift," I told him.

"I told you that you can do it," he said. At this point, I realized I was dreaming, and then I realized that the dream was actually a recollection of my conversation in the past with the psychic surgeon.

"You also told me others can do it as well, so there really is no pressure for me," I said.

"Yes, but you are different," he said.

My answer in the dream then became opposite of what I told him way back.

"That is true," I said. "I want to be an artist, not a psychic surgeon. I tell people I'm weird, but I only go that far. I am already, in a sense, an outcast now, but if I do what you do, I will really become the outcast I claim myself to be."

It was like an updated answer. Why did I say "outcast"?

He appeared to be speaking some more. I tried to listen, but I wasn't hearing anything. Then I woke up.

ಏ

When I came to the United States, I began forgetting names. I can remember names of some old classmates and many of my friends my age, but I can't remember the names of my teachers anymore, except for maybe five.

Let's say I spent five years in the United States in a state of culture shock and psychological adjustment. Let's say that by 1992, I began attempting to recall people's name, including this psychic surgeon, whom I considered a mentor, but whose ways and abilities shocked me.

It was only in 2006 that his first name came back to me. I still cannot remember his last name. I can remember his smiling, friendly face. I must admit, I miss him. He had such an impact on me.

I chose to forget his name to keep my sanity. It was only now that can I talk about my experiences, at a time when horror movies, documentaries about ghosts, and my own dreams of my dead relatives no longer scared me. It had been twenty years in 2006 as I wrote this chapter for the original memoir that I pulled out of circulation. It has been twenty-eight years as I attempt to publish this chapter and the rest of this book in 2014.

☙

I remember having a hard time finding his home that first Sunday I showed up. It took me at least three jeepney rides to get there, plus a few minutes of walking.

He lived in a more congested place in the city. A lot more children were playing in the streets, and the road in front of his house seemed to be newly cemented. In Manila, a newly paved road that showed no clues of previous paving meant that it was only recently that the local politicians noticed the neighborhood, most probably because it was a poorer section of the metropolis.

I came late, about twenty minutes before the service was to begin. I was supposed to be there an hour before service. A girl introduced herself as a daughter of the healer. I asked to use the bathroom and excused myself.

In the bathroom, as I peed, I noticed a red plastic container with a handle. It was on the window pane, the window being an open square foot, with a cheap plastic curtain. There was a big barrel with an open top filled almost to the brim with water. I figured they fetched water from somewhere. The red container was used to scoop water from the barrel, to fill up the bigger pail next to the toilet, for flushing, and for taking a bath.

There's a joke about bathing in the Philippines.

"Where's the tub?" the foreigner asks.

"Tub? Oh tab! Here! Tah-bo... *Tabo!*" answered the Filipino, handing a container the size of the red plastic. "Wash yourself with the tabo!"

Tabo is a Filipino word for "mug." When used for bathing, it refers more for a gigantic mug or a container for scooping water, with or without a handle, with just the right, sensible amount of water to pour on the head. Just enough so as not to waste fetched water.

When I came back out, he was there.

He said hello, offered me something to drink, and then took me to another room, the kitchen, where we sat on old, wooden, homemade stools, next to the folding laminate table, the only table in there.

He started, "I'm a psychic surgeon, and you have to understand the basis of all these that we do. We believe in God and Jesus Christ. We are Christians, but a lot of us are no longer Catholic."

"Why not?" I asked.

"Well, we hold our own service here at home, for example, and I don't go to church anymore. I'm supposed to be the leader of this group. I'm married. You've met my children outside.

"I'm not going to convert you to my beliefs, but I will show passages from the Bible which support psychic surgery," he explained.

The psychic surgeon reached for a well-used Bible with plenty of pen marks and a few bookmarks. He pointed to a familiar passage in the Bible. Genesis.

He read it, "I am the Alpha and the Omega." Then he paused a little.

Continuing, he said, "Think about this, Val. Even in grade school, we were taught that God is omnipresent, omniscient, and omnipotent.

"We live in linear time. You know, we are born, then in time we get older and older. God isn't like that. God exists in the past, the present, and the future. Time is nothing to God. And the only way for Him to achieve this is to be omnipresent, omniscient, and omnipotent. In order for people in the past to understand this, God simply stated that He is the First and the Last, and everything in between.

"He is the Alpha and the Omega, while we exist only in the middle of the First and the Last. This means that we can make decisions on our own. Whatever we decide on, it would not divert from God, because He started everything His way. No matter what we do in the middle, it will still be God's will that will end everything.

"This means that we can empower ourselves to live our lives the way we want it to be.

"Being that I am a faith healer, I would ask God to change the life of a person for the better. If a person is sick, then I would ask God to change the course of that person, and ask God to heal the person.

"A person can die today or ten years from today, and God's plan to make the final decision would not be affected. So we might as well ask for healing! He wouldn't mind!" He said that with a smile.

☙

While you're reading this, I'm going to talk crazy. It's my book anyway.

To me, now that I'm writing this, extrapolating from what the man said, everything is One.

This is where my mathematics comes in. How I feel God

works mathematically.

In math, there's geometry, algebra, trigonometry, and all that fun stuff. Especially in high school, everything was compartmentalized that way. It felt as if they were separate fields.

Three years after my encounter with the psychic surgeon, and still recovering from the "eyeopener," I went for my masters degree in Actuarial Science, which was applied math. I was introduced to serious calculus.

It seemed to appear to me, that all the equations are just ways to interpret space and volume, "pinched" from a whole, three-dimensional "One."

Then I got into analyzing mathematical series, which also seemed to approach that single "One."

Physics and other sciences seemed to approach the same concept of "One."

It is like watching an explosion in chemistry class, which involved physics, which involved math.

I think that "One" is God. That all the sciences do bear witness to God.

I was really impacted by the experience with the psychic surgeon. And then three years later, Mathematics reminded me of God. Crazy talk.

☙

The psychic surgeon continued.

"When someone dies, he goes to rejoin God.

"The same concept can be seen in the Big Bang Theory of the creation of the universe. Everything was as one, then thanks to the Big Bang, things became compartmentalized into stars and planets and whatever else is out there.

"Looking at the earth, everything continues to be separated into land, air, and water, animals and plants and microorganisms, each segregated further all the way down to various species, then down to tissues and organs, cells, molecules, and atoms.

"When something expands, it will eventually contract. Everything will collapse back to return to the Source, which is God. When someone dies, the soul rejoins God.

"I believe that hell remains for those souls who cannot accept losing their consciousness, when rejoining with God after they die. That will be hell.

"Hell happens for those people who do not want to rejoin God's Oneness. They continue to want to steer away.

"Heaven is the same nature of joining with God. However, this time, the joining is accepted. To rejoin God, that will be the ultimate experience and discovery. That will be heaven," he said. Lengthy. I was confused.

"How does all this play in the healing?" I asked.

He continued, smiling. "First, the Oneness, as far as a single person is concerned, can be realized through perfect health. Disease can be a distraction from the Oneness with God, if you let it.

"I still don't understand," I said.

"Bear with me, you came here to know what I have to say. Let me continue. I know that all this is a lot to bear in one afternoon, so I will ask you to come back a few more times. But for now, let me continue, take notes, and you will understand me later on.

"By accepting that we still belong to God's Oneness, even while currently compartmentalized, then it just follows that God's healing power can be tapped to make a person healthy and one with Him again.

While we were still in the kitchen, the psychic surgeon showed me another verse in the New Testament.

He said, "Here is something where Christ said that if you want to communicate with God, go to your room, and there you can speak with Him."

He continued, "So, I ask you, what if you're on a train, and there are no rooms? What if you need to talk to God at that time? How can you do it? It doesn't make sense to stop the train, and try to find a room that you would be comfortable in, right?

"The room Christ was talking about was the mind. If you closed your eyes and asked to be with God, that is your room. That is where you can ask for healing or intervention.

"So it would mean that if you concentrated all the time, and imagined being with God, it would improve your psychic abilities. Eventually, you can become a psychic surgeon if you want to go that route," he finished.

"The first lesson stated that we should acknowledge the given end, that we will be one with God in the end.

"The next lesson makes the assumption that whatever we do now is temporary anyway, and will not affect the end. Therefore, God will allow what we want to happen. A healer can therefore ask for healing.

"Knowing such outcomes in the long term, a psychic surgeon like me has deduced that God will allow us to alter what is current and temporary. In terms of health, if we are sick, God will allow us to be healthy.

"Look at me again," he said, as he brought his head up, looking into my eyes more seriously. "The people come to me for healing, thinking that I am so connected with God, that I am so near God. But look around you. I am poor. My kitchen is not the best you've seen."

"The people here think that I am their leader, because they think I do miraculous things. Here I am telling you, I'm just in a temporary, present situation, with the ability to ask God to heal people who wanted to be healed.

"This last lesson is about being with God, in the present time. The way to do it is by closing your eyes and visualizing being in His presence.

"Then you acknowledge that God is already in you. The ability to heal is already in you. Then it's just a matter of tapping into what you already have. It's all in the mind and a matter of perception," he said, smiling. He was relaxed as he explained all this. He had charisma. He made me listen.

I was listening, but I was also amused at the same time. My term paper was taking shape.

"I think we should continue another day," he said finishing his talk. I said thanks, and he led me out of the kitchen and into the front, bigger room. His service was delayed because of me. There were probably about thirty people already waiting for him.

Some people came to us, and I was introduced to the regulars—people who come over not for healing, but for worship. For lack of a better word, they were his followers.

The psychic surgeon came to the table that was in the front and center of the room. The table's rectangular shape and size were familiar. This was where he did his healing on.

He stood in front of it and spoke first.

He said that everyone should be reminded that this was a gathering in God's Name. He reminded everyone, mentioning that he had said it weekly, to acknowledge that whatever healing that took place, that night and in the future, it was not done by him, but by God. He was just an instrument.

The way he explained, I thought, sounded redundant, much like the way he explained things to me in the kitchen. I looked at the people who were listening. It did seem that they needed more sentences.

A couple of sentences welcomed me, and indicated that I was observing for a school paper.

Then he asked for the first patient. The patient, a lady, laid down on the table. He talked to her for a while, then he put his hands on her stomach and exposed her belly.

I saw his fingers go through the skin.

He asked me to come closer. He lifted his hands and showed me an open hole.

Smiling, he told me that the patient did not feel any pain, because the "power of God" was overwhelmingly powerful enough to be an anesthetic.

He also said that he didn't wear any gloves, because the healing session, being in the realm of God, also had an antiseptic effect.

For lack of any scientific study or further analysis of tissues, I saw him take out what I thought were blood clots from the lady's stomach. He placed them on some tissue paper, next to a red container that had some water in it. Then he dipped his hands into the red container.

I recognized the container. It was the same container I saw in the bathroom! He wiped his hands dry on a white towel and then his hands went back into the wound. He did this a few more times.

Then he closed the wound by placing his right hand flat on the opening. When he lifted it, the wound was gone! It was not so much like magic as much as it reminded me of the awe when I was a child watching a magic trick. There was a difference.

He proceeded to "treat" other patients.

Several times, on occasion, he closed his eyes and concentrated. Sometimes he seemed to pray, chant, or cast a spell. His mouth moved, but he was silent.

He told me later, he was praying to God.

I left for home, that night. I came back the following Sunday.

☙

2014 update. When the psychic surgeon said, "The room Christ was talking about was the mind," I distinctly remember what he did, which in 2006, I paid no attention to, so I did not write about it.

He closed his eyes, bowed his head a little as, his hand rose from the Bible to meet his head, and with his right forefinger, he pointed to the center of his forehead.

I had never heard about the pineal gland until 2012. On YouTube, I saw people discuss the pineal gland, pointing to the same exact spot this healer did decades ago.

It's just a commonality I want to point out.

If you think about it, when talking about the intellect in an informal manner, people point to the side of their heads. However, this man and everyone who talked about the pineal gland, in all seriousness, pointed to the center of their foreheads.

If you are not yet familiar with the pineal gland, you might want to look at some videos on YouTube, for starters, then research about it on your own. Riddles!

Chapter 35

Lessons from a Psychic Surgeon 2

Once again, I was late. This time we agreed for me to stay later, so he can administer to the patients on time.

By the time the group dwindled, and there were no more "patients" who needed healing, the afternoon had gotten dark.

The man spent varied lengths of time with the patients. I guessed it depended on what his instincts told him.

☙

We sat by the kitchen table again, in the next room.

He talked.

"I have done visualization healing before, too. Like one time, a sick person was far away, the family simply sent me a photograph."

"Did it work?" I asked.

"I would say that the person felt better," he answered.

"I always ask for people to go to their medical doctors first. It's not always a good thing to come to a psychic healer."

I asked, "When do you advocate going to psychic healers, then?"

He answered, "When you're poor—because we don't charge—you can come over. Or when the doctors couldn't find out what's wrong with you.

"There are also bad spirits, for example, which can make you sick. Like the effects of bad witchcraft or possession by a bad spirit.

"Or like one of my followers, the one who is clinically blind. If he wanted to see again, I could help him. Christ was able to make the blind see; you have to believe that that's possible."

I was still trying to comprehend the witchcraft part. "You've seen witchcraft and possession?" I asked.

"Yeah, you stay here long enough and you'll see it, too," he answered.

I chuckled a little. "I'm not so sure I can deal with that. I'm just here for my term paper. Make the grade and graduate. I'll show up a few more times, though."

He said, "Okay. Put it this way then. Do you know that my organization alone lists at least 150 psychic surgeons in the Philippines? Compare that to only one or two people who can do the same thing elsewhere. Don't you find that weird?

"There's something special about the Philippines, you know. Something psychic or supernatural. At the same token that this happens among Filipinos, you can make a guess that other things happen here as well, like maybe there are other invisible forces or spirits in our midst.

"Well, even the concept of God is a mystery," he continued. "Based on what the Bible says, you really don't have to understand God to ask Him for help. That's where faith comes in.

"We can go on and on about many things and arrive at the same place we started. Let's just go back to psychic surgery," he said, grabbing the Bible that was next to him.

୪୨

Opening the Bible to a bookmarked page, the psychic surgeon pointed at a passage:

"When two or more people are gathered in My Name, there I am in the midst of them."

"Think about this passage," he said. "Once again, be reminded that I'm not the healer, Jesus Christ is, and if you expand it some more, God is. I'm just the instrument through which the healing power of Christ passes. This is why it is important for the group to meet."

"Christ guarantees in this passage that He will definitely be present if there are more than just one person together. It has to be a group. So if you think about it, if my group is gathered around, I am assured that Christ is nearby and can be contacted for healing. I can therefore ask Christ, or God, for healing energy. Of course we can ask for other things."

"But I've read that passage before!" I said.

"Yes, so this time, you return to the passage with the point of view of a psychic surgeon. You acknowledge that there is a psychic link between you and Christ, and tap into that power so you can do what I can do."

൚

I asked, "What about the allegation of mass hypnosis coming into the picture? People allege that psychic healers hypnotize the group to believe that psychic surgery takes place. Something about hypnotic suggestions."

"Yes, people can keep saying that," he said, "except that you've seen me work. You've seen up close that the skin does open up, and I am able to place my hand, not just fingers, into the open skin, especially if the opening is on the belly."

"All this scares me," I told him. "It would be nice if I can heal people, but I'm really not ready to get my hands into people that way."

"What about infection? Don't your patients get infected?" I asked.

"Not at all," he answered. "No one gets infected. When God wants people to heal, you have to believe that the healing power radiates like a ball of light, encompassing everything. The sphere will not allow for infection from outside sources. Everything is clean."

I commented, "I have to be honest with you. That red container the size of a saucepan, the one that you used, was in the bathroom when I first came in. It's probably the same one your daughter used when she took a bath. Then, you used it to wash your bare hands in as you did psychic surgery on the people. Don't you think you should use something else?"

"Well," he said, motioning around the room, "there's really nothing else here that we can use, don't you agree? Besides, we all believe that during the healing sessions, and all throughout the time we all get together, in the name of God, everything is cleansed. You have to believe that."

∞

He looked back at the Bible. "Once again, Christ said, 'Where there are two or more people gathered in My Name, there I am in the midst of them.' So if Christ is there, or here, why can't you see Him?

"Remember that Christ used to be human, but not anymore. You really cannot visualize His present state, because He's God, just like the Father.

"So I have this visualization exercise. I concentrate and in my mind, I pray:

"Christ, I know that You are God, and that You are no longer human, but please for this healing session, appear to me in human form," he said.

"What happens?" I asked.

He explained, "It's a visual aid. I see Christ in my imagination based on the religious images that we have all seen. Then I open my eyes and I see Him as a human being smiling at me in the room. I then let this visualized Christ guide me."

"How are you guided?" I asked.

"I sometimes see Christ put His hands on the patient, effecting healing, or sometimes I see Him directing me to put my hands on the patient.

"Sometimes I feel like I have to place my hands on the feet of the patient, then go to the head and then touch the head. Sometimes, I touch the shoulders, the hands, or the stomach. It's all like a progression of where to touch the person based on how I feel, but to better aid me in doing this, I let my imagined Christ guide me."

I asked, "That works?"

"It's been a technique I've been doing right from the start. Whether it works or not, I can't say, but you really have to look at all this in a wholistic way.

"It's hard to explain which part works and which is imaginary. Why don't you try it?" he asked.

I asked back, "What do you mean?"

"Close your eyes," he requested.

I closed my eyes.

"Now tell yourself, silently, in your mind, Christ please appear to me in human form," he said.

I told myself the phrase.

He asked, "What do you see?"

I answered, "I see Christ in the way He is portrayed in paintings."

"That's the Christ I want you to see. Now when you open your eyes, imagine that His image has not left. Imagine that you continue to see Him standing somewhere in the room," he said.

I opened my eyes. Then I said, "Okay I see him in the corner of the room."

"Okay, now all you have to do is to let Christ do what He wills, either as Himself or through you," he said.

"So that's how you touch people?" I asked.

"Yes," he answered.

☙

"Have you ever touched people and you felt it was inappropriate? You know what I mean?" I asked.

"Of course not!" he exclaimed. Then he laughed. "You must understand something. If you're talking about sex, I do have sex with my wife. However, it is a known fact amongst psychic healers that there is need for religion and values. There is need for meditation and connection with Christ and God, in order to heal.

"We have observed that sex dissipates the healing energy. Bad intentions also dissipate healing energy. You have to be pure in thought.

"There is something else that you must take into consideration."

"What?" I asked.

"That evil will follow you if you are doing the mission of spreading God's Word," he said.

"So you'd be giving in to evil by having improper thoughts?" I asked.

"Not just that," he nodded. "Evil itself can attack you when you are vulnerable. This means that you have to be on guard, always."

"So inappropriate touching is bad," I concluded.

"It's bad not because your patient might slap you in the face; it's worse than that," he said.

"When you have a person coming to you for healing, you are already committed to gathering in God's Name. That means evil is not far behind.

"The moment that you are in a healing session, that moment is like the apex of the event. That is the moment when you cannot afford to have impure thoughts and inappropriate touching. Your intention to be in touch with God and to heal is also built up to that moment. Therefore, there can be no room for bad thoughts at all. Not before, not during and not after the healing sessions.

"So inappropriate touching or improper thoughts, or even thoughts that occur to you that are not needed in the healing process are not just inadvisable; they have to be avoided altogether," he explained.

"Okay," I agreed.

"Continuing with the visualization exercise. When you touch or lay your hands on a person for healing, you must imagine a transfer of positive healing energy.

"When you are dealing with a person whom you suspect is evil or is influenced by evil, or if you think is possessed by the devil, then you must go further by imagining the transfer of God Himself. Or you imagine another type of energy that is stronger than physical healing," he explained.

"You imagine energy rays or something?" I asked.

He explained, "Well, the easiest way to imagine energy transfer is imagining the energy in the form of light. For example, if you imagine white healing light coming from yourself to the patient, that would be good."

"Okay, so the imaginary light contains the healing energy?" I said.

"Right," he answered. "You've seen me holding my palms above a patient sometimes."

"Yes," I said. "I remember."

"You might also see my fingers pointing to the patient, like a magician," he said. "Sometimes, I imagine healing rays coming from my palms, when I feel like doing that, and sometimes I imagine healing rays coming from my fingers.

"Then, sometimes I feel that the time is right for the skin to open up.

"For example, if the person complains of a stomach ache, then there is tension in the stomach. It could be ulcers for example. So I point to the ulcer, and that's when the skin opens up, and I'm able to penetrate the skin and perform psychic surgery. I place my hand inside, and if I feel there's something that is loose, then I take it out. Usually it's a blood clot."

I asked, "What is it sometimes?"

He paused and looked at me sternly. "Don't get spooked if

you want to hear more," he said. And he laughed.

To be continued... Suspenseful music.

CHAPTER 36

LESSONS FROM A PSYCHIC SURGEON 3

"Okay," I told him. "I'm ready to get more scared. What have you pulled out of people's stomachs so far?"

"I've pulled out worms. You know, parasites. Then there have been times, but very rarely, when other objects came out."

"Like what?" I asked.

He asked, "Remember when I said that a lot of people who come to me are desperate and have unexplainable illnesses?"

"Yeah?"

He continued, "There was a time when I pulled out locks of hair from a lady's stomach. Then some bugs came out. She was so horrified, my followers had to hold her."

"How do you explain that?" I asked.

"Some type of *kulam*. It turned out, she was the mistress of another woman's husband. The real wife was so mad she went to ask for help from someone who did kulam," he explained.

Filipinos, for lack of a better word, would say that *kulam*, pronounced "KOO-lam," directly means witchcraft. I don't think that's an accurate translation anymore. Kulam is more the visualization of bad intentions, with the intention of inflicting harm on an individual.

There is a word in the Philippines that also has a vague literal translation, or spelling even—*espiritista*, or *ispiritista*, referring to a person. "Spiritist," in English, has more to do with someone who communicates with the dead. *Espiritista* has more to do with someone who has a religious slant on things, and uses it, either for healing (faith healing), ritual, praying, visualizations and maybe even exorcism.

"So you can attest that kulam is real?" I asked.

"Psychic surgery is real, and it still cannot be explained. Like I said, it's all about the mind, and visualization, and faith in God and the unknown. Some people take it another way, and with bad intentions," he said.

"Is kulam easy?" I asked.

"Kulam is as easy as psychic surgery, if you can believe that. It's just that there's a different set of underlying beliefs," he explained.

"Evil?" I asked.

"Not necessarily evil. Bad intentions and grudges are easy to have in people. And then there is ignorance, desperation and fascination," he added.

"What do you mean?" I asked.

"Imagine that you are poor and uneducated. Then you discover that you can have visualization techniques that can result in inflicting damage. Then people come to you for it. It would appear that you have found your purpose in life. You become a *mangkukulam*. (A person who practices kulam.)

"Bad intentions that result in strange outcomes is misuse of God's power, with the help of evil spirits.

"I think here is a lie from the devil," he said.

I asked, "What is?"

He continued, "That people think that the devil has powers. You should know that whatever powers the devil has, they are actually powers that come from God. They are not even powers allowed by God. They are God's.

"So the devil is deceiving people into thinking that he also has powers that are the exact opposite of God's, and of what I do. That's the way I put it together.

"It's not a matter of overpowering the devil, it's just a matter of taking the power away from the devil because that power is yours and God's to begin with."

"That's a different perspective," I said, "but does it work?"

"It works for me," he answered.

※

"Moving along, when you begin to visualize healing, here is an easy way to visualize healing rays.

"Imagine that heaven is in a room just a few feet above you and the patient. Imagine opening up the clouds of heaven, or however you see heaven, at will, and imagine the light coming down and enveloping your patient.

"Sometimes you imagine opening it up to only the diseased area, or sometimes you imagine the entire body getting covered in healing light.

"If you feel that the person is possessed, you must imagine a different kind of light. It will not be healing light touching the person anymore, but God Himself.

"Then again, you can imagine that it is God Himself as rays of light touching the person, even when the person is physically diseased.

"It's all how you feel you should go about," he said.

"So bring heaven down to the person? Or God down to the person?" I asked.

"Yes, well, we're talking about seeing the person as still being on earth.

"Sometimes you would try to visualize bringing the person to heaven," he said.

"How is that?" I asked.

"Have you ever heard of psychic projection?" he asked. "Or astral projection? That sometimes your soul or mind is able to leave your physical body?"

He continued, "Let's assume that is possible, not counting my belief system, for the sake of argument. People have claimed that such a thing has occurred before.

"I try to visualize the patient, but this time, I try to visualize the soul or the astral body going up to heaven, just a few feet from the body. Or sometimes I visualize that I raise the entire body, including the physical body up into heaven for healing." He then shifted the topic a little.

☙

"When I did an exorcism, I visualized God himself entering the body of the patient in all levels I can imagine—physical, spiritual, astral, mental, in order to get the evil spirit away.

"It was like I was just trying to displace the spirit.

"Then I visualized a protective aura around the person so the evil could not come back," he said.

"It worked?" I asked.

"You have to trust your instincts. Your instincts will tell you if a patient will have to keep coming back for a few more times for the exorcism to be complete. Sometimes it can't be done in just a single session. I also ask for the laying on of hands by other believers, which is where the rest of this congregation comes in. They help me out. At the place where you met me the first time, if more than one psychic surgeon or psychic healer is needed, especially at times when the patient seemed affected by some bad force, then we all help out and heal together."

(When we were conversing in Filipino, my questions did not seem out of place, skeptical and doubtful. This interview is a recollection of my past conversations with the psychic surgeon. The message is all his, but I had to reorganize and translate everything into English. Some flavors do get lost in translation.)

"How can you tell that a person is possessed?" I asked him further.

"I pray, and I can sense it, but I have a way to let the evil make itself known for other people to see," he said.

"How?" I asked.

"I concentrate and pray even before a healing service. By the time I'm doing my healing sessions, suffice it to say that I'm fully energized with the power from God," he said.

He continued, "I concentrate God's energy to a hand, like my right hand for example. Then I take the hand of the person, and I press one finger, or hold the entire hand, imagining a transfer of God Himself. A possessed person would react, sometimes scream in pain, even with just a light touch of the finger."

"That would be one way? Or are there any more ways?"

He answered, "Some healers use other ways. You know how some old folks use eggs to divine evil or transfer evil and then there are some who use pendulums? I do those things, sometimes, when I feel like it. Did you see me try to divine the patient's condition with white bond paper and water?"

I answered, "Yeah, earlier, I noticed you prayed over the water, and touched the patient with the container. Then you dipped the paper into the water and held it afterwards against the light. You showed the paper to me, and I did not see anything. I was going to ask you about that."

"I used my instincts and judged the person from that paper," he said. "I usually see some type of a sign on it."

"Does it always work?" I asked.

"Well, in time you learn to decipher the blotches. Sometimes I notice something really different. You just need to get used to all this."

"That's not very scientific," I told him.

He agreed. "No, it's not. But it works for me. There's no science to all of this. At least not yet. Some foreign researchers have actually come to the Philippines to observe me and a lot of others. I've shown you photographs of researchers coming over.

"I myself had flown out of the country, paid for by convinced people who wanted me to do healing sessions where their friends and contacts were, but at the end of the day, there would just be my teachings and photographs of my hand and an open, gaping would.

"My beliefs and underlying principles can be documented but cannot be proven.

"Then I really do all this on the weekend. I have to work too, you know. We're always pressed for time. There's not enough time to prove things that are abstract."

"Yeah, I realize that there is no way for you to prove this, or for you to leave your work and your family so you can be with scientists who can document what you can do," I said.

"Right," he said, "and besides, it is rare, for example, that someone comes to me cursed by a mangkukulam or possessed by some evil entity.

℘

"Let's talk again about how strange the Philippines is, having 150 Filipino psychic surgeons.

"Here in the Philippines—just imagine this—more than 150 psychic surgeons belong to my association. Add to this the fact that there is also an even bigger number of people who are not psychic surgeons, but psychic healers or faith healers. Other countries do not have this many psychic surgeons. Or healers," he said.

I asked him, "Where are you leading this to?"

"It means that there must be a lot of unseen forces here in our country. Start with the notion that there might be different levels of existence here. There is us, humans, and you have heard of elves, right?"

I answered, "Dwarfs? They're supposed to be invisible to humans unless they decide to show themselves?"

"That's right," he said. "Elves or dwarfs or dwarves. And then there are ghosts. Then there are ogres and all those other mythical beings, which just might not be mythical at all."

A memory struck me then.

"Oh yeah," I said, "in Bataan, where my grandmother was born, they have a place that they call Balon Anito, which sort of means Well of Enchanted Spirits."

I continued, "They have this story, that after the Liberation, after World War II, the American soldiers were running into the town all panicked, wet and naked. They claimed to have seen a *kapre* (pronounced "KAHP-reh"). They said that in the distance, they saw this really dark-skinned giant with huge red eyes, atop a tree, smoking a cigar, and he was looking at them. They were bathing in the river and the kapre scared them."

"Based on the stories we hear to begin with," he added, other beings don't necessarily have to be evil, just because they are invisible. People say that, sometimes, a person gets ill because that person was affected by an invisible being. For example, we hear of stories of sick people with undiagnosed illnesses, who recollected that they probably started getting sick after peeing in the woods in the dark.

"I have been able to make people get back to normal, by my own attempts to appease some invisible entity. It's the same thing with kulam. Kulam involves people, but people are not purely evil.

"Of course all this is a matter of perceiving things, but I had a patient who claimed that he saw a dwarf appear to him before he got sick."

I sat back in my chair and shook my head. "Wow. Now that I'm hearing all this, it seems that through psychic surgery and psychic healing, I'm bound to encounter all of this scary stuff. Going to medical school is sounding better and better already."

He smiled at me. "You know, if I can only afford to go to medical school, I would have done it already.

"To be honest, my efforts in healing stemmed from my own, personal search for meaning. There was a time when I was so depressed, I seemed unable to move forward with my own life.

"I took some time off my work, and stayed at home for the most part. I went to a psychic healer to see what was going on with me.

"I then read the Bible, looking for guidance and passages that could be relevant to my life. That was when a revelation came to me, that I can probably become a psychic healer.

"It took me years to do psychic surgery myself, but even before that, I already had formed a group for healing and Bible readings, and we were already meeting weekly. At the same time, I also joined the group of Christian Spiritists, and where I met other people who were able to do this as well."

☙

I asked, "Has anyone died in your hands? Has anyone gotten infected?"

"Infected, no," he answered.

"You don't wear gloves," I said.

"I have never worn gloves," he said. "I believe that by the time my hands can affect healing, they become protected. I become protected from infection, and my patients are protected from infection from my hands as well."

"What if you wore gloves?"

He answered, "I can wear gloves if I had any. It will not change what I can do."

"So healing energy is not diminished by rubber gloves? Not like electricity?" I asked.

He answered, "No. Right now, I'm skilled enough with psychic surgery that I don't even have to touch the skin to make it open up. I can wave my hand as distant as a foot away from the patient, or even more, and the skin would continue to be receptive. It will open up.

"Maybe it's not just power generated by me, but the intention of the patient to get healed, plus the intent to heal by rest of the group, all this makes certain things possible.

☙

"Let me tell you something else," he continued.

"There had been a couple of times when someone recently died, and was brought to me. I was able to revive them."

"How do you explain that?" I asked.

"This is a poor community that I live in. People cannot really see doctors on a regular basis. So someone at one time got a heart attack, and he was brought to me supposedly already dead. But the person supposedly just died, so his body was not decomposed. Then again, maybe he was just unconscious, right? So I can't really say that mine is a proven method."

"What's the method?" I asked.

"I laid down next to the dead person, and I astral projected. I saw myself getting out of my body, and I imagined going to heaven or where the person was. I visualized talking to the person to come back to his body. The person revived and I came back to my own body," he said.

"In just a few minutes?" I asked.

He explained, "No, I didn't notice the time pass, but it took a really long time. That one took eight hours. It was like I was asleep next to the person.

"I realized that the next time I did that, I should probably also imagine that my physical body was protected from evil and other entities, just so no other spirit goes in my physical body while I'm away. I also realized, that if I am to revive a dead person, I should do some visualizing where the body of the person also does not decompose. Remember these are all just my theories. I can't prove it, and it's not like I had the chance to do this everyday.

"The second chance a supposedly dead, maybe comatose person was brought to me, I had in my mind the theory that decomposition probably happens when the soul is not in the body.

"I imagined my own being inhabiting the body of the person that was placed next to me, at the same time imagining being where the person's soul was, and convincing the person to come back to his own body. The person revived.

"Obviously I cannot recommend this to anyone. I actually hope this does not happen to me all the time. However, my daughter can tell you she had also done this once. I was away when someone was brought here. The trouble with this is that it is hard to prove and everything is just my speculation."

"Your daughter was able to do it?" I asked.

There was an air of confidence in his answer. "Of course, whatever I have told you, I have told everyone."

He continued, "My daughter has heard all this. Then she tried to do it, obviously because I was not around. Out of desperation—the need was there."

I asked him then, "Is this supported by the Bible?"

"Yes," he answered. "It's in the story of Lazarus. Christ came back to Lazarus' town only to discover that Lazarus had died. You should analyze that story."

"How?"

"To begin with, Lazarus had died. Maybe it was really time for him to die. But why would Christ bring him back? Maybe simply to prove His powers? Also, remember that before Christ was able to revive Lazarus, Christ wept?

"Christ weeping—could it mean that Christ lamented because He Himself wasn't sure that Lazarus was going to revive anyway? Thankfully, he revived. Then again, if Christ failed, it might not be included in the Bible anyway, at least not in the way it was told. So, if Christ was sure to revive him, he did not have to weep. So it might happen or it might not happen. In my two cases, yes, I was able to revive the persons, but maybe they were really just unconscious to begin with," he said.

"You have no documentation?" I asked.

"Would you rather have the persons in question sign written statements that they died and got rejuvenated?"

I laughed.

"You should also remember, there is a part in the Bible where it is said that the dead will walk amongst the living. So somehow you must accept that this is possible.

"My belief made me be able to do what I did. I just used it in my own situation," he said.

I commented, "The way you explain it, you seem to have your own doubts."

He smiled. "Well, I'm talking to you, right?"

"What about me?" I asked.

"Your educational background is science. I am telling you what I have to say in a way that you might receive it or accept it in a more logical way.

ఇ

"Going back to the idea of God, that He is all-knowing, all-seeing, and all-powerful, as I have mentioned in the first place, I forgot to let you know that you can actually learn three more specific lessons from that.

"From the concept of being all-powerful, you can tap God's power to effect healing power.

"From the concept of being all-knowing, you can tap into God's power to diagnose an illness or get a general idea of the person.

"From the concept of being all-seeing is the concept of being everywhere.

"This third one means that a psychic surgeon or healer does not have to be in front of the patient to heal the patient. Distance need not be an object.

"There was a time when someone claimed she saw me somewhere, when I was actually someplace else," he said.

"What do you mean?" I asked.

"I was in Manila, but someone wrote to me for healing and the person was in another location. I concentrated and visualized that I was near the person, and another person that same day claimed that she saw me near the sick person's house.

"It could not have been a dream because she was outside the house. Maybe it was someone else she saw, but the person claimed that I was there. So there are still things which even I have yet to discover," he said.

I asked, "Has that ever happened again?"

"No," he said, "so it could be a fluke, but then again, I do entertain impossible things in my mind, whether or not you are able to accept it. It is my own world that I make."

"You seem to have such great faith, you leave everything to belief," I said.

"That is true. We are what we decide and perceive for ourselves. All this works well for me, and I don't really take time to prove myself right or wrong. I just go ahead and if it works, then it works; if it does not, then it does not. But I maintain my faith. That would be the constant," he said.

"So it could be because of your faith that you allow for the impossible to happen?" I asked.

"That's right," he said. "But claiming it to be faith just leaves nothing much for science and fact."

"Well," I told him, "you have told me a lot. My term paper is taking shape, but it will not be as scientific as I thought. It will tackle the experience of being with you. It will be objective in the sense that I will tell your teachings as sort of a story, all coming from you. It will be a documentation of what you yourself are claiming. I will be quoting you a lot."

He agreed. "Sounds like a good way to approach it."

I was to see him again the following week.

Chapter 37

Lessons from a Psychic Surgeon 4

"I want to tell you about the power of words," said the psychic surgeon.

"What do you mean?" I asked.

"I want to tell you the time when it rained so hard that my companions and I should have gotten wet" he asked.

"What's the story?" I asked.

He narrated, "One late afternoon, we were going somewhere, and it rained so suddenly. It poured. By instinct I said something, and my intention was for us not to get wet. Guess what? We did not get wet."

"How did that happen?" I asked matter-of-factly.

"I think it was the intention. The intention was there, and I uttered something, like a single word, and when we got to the house, we were not wet! But I'm still figuring this incident out," he said.

He asked, "When you make your term paper on psychic surgery and psychic healing, what do you hope it will accomplish?"

"I want it to be meaningful and well-written, so I can get a good grade," I said.

"Right, but there should be more to it than that," he added.

"Well, I want it to connect with the reader," I said.

"So there is a connection that you hope to gain. What is the magnitude of that connection?" he asked.

"What do you mean?" I asked back.

"Well, who will read your work?" he asked

"Probably just my teacher," I answered.

He asked, "What if other people read your work?"

I answered, "If others read it, then it must be readable for them as well. Plus I must be responsible, from the start, to have reported it correctly, whether one person reads it, or the entire university."

He asked, "Doesn't that mean that once you wrote your term paper, then you accept responsibility for your work, whether one person reads it or a million people read it?"

"I would not say that," I answered.

"What do you mean?" he asked.

I explained, "Well the reader is also responsible for what he reads and takes in. So the interaction remains between the writer and the reader. Hopefully 50-50. The writer is responsible, and the reader is responsible.

"Then again, if I made a textbook on brain surgery, just because the how-to information is there does not mean anyone can hold the book in front of him and operate on a brain. The reader has to be smart enough. It takes time to read, but longer to learn," I laughed.

Then I asked, "So what does that have to do with what you were saying earlier?"

"Well, I may not write as well as you, but going back to that one incident with the rain—that night, one word to connect with God was enough for us not to get wet. So, since I believe that everything stems from God, the connection was with God, and He proceeded to not get us wet," he said.

"I really find that hard to believe," I said. I was becoming a little more comfortable with his presence, I told my peace.

"I understand you will say that, but I am just telling you that this event occurred and I will be looking into it some more," he said.

"Did that happen again?" I asked.

"No, I'm still trying to figure out how it happened," he said.

"Can you experiment and see if it happens again?" I asked.

He answered, "Well, it was spontaneous, but there's something that came to me then. That words can be powerful. You, for example, are writing a term paper. You are documenting what I have to say. You don't need a miracle to realize the power that your words can have."

"It's just a term paper," I said with humility.

"Right, you're saying it's just words, but you don't know who will read it," he said.

I said, "My teacher will read it. Then it goes to the library, and I don't know who will read it. Not unless my teacher decides to keep it in her office."

"She likes your writing?" he asked.

I beamed. I said, "I have shown potential. My dad sent me, my brother and my sister to a speedreading school, about 2 years ago. After that I was able to read a lot faster. The school, through the course, forced us to read a lot of books. When I got out of there, I came to a realization that there are so many books to be read, so little time. I came to respect writers.

"Then I realized that I can be a writer myself if I want. After that, I used my English and Filipino classes with writing assignments to get better. In a short time, the teachers started reading my works in class. But I'm a very shy person, and I was just glad that they did not identify me to my classmates. I thought it was embarrassing to be identified. I didn't realize that I can be a good writer. I just wrote what was in my heart, in a more honest manner and then tried to be objective and ordered. I did my best to progress logically with my ideas, and put them on paper."

"So you got embarrassed?" he asked.

I said, "Getting praised and getting identified are two separate things. The teachers praised me without the need to identify me. So reading my writing in my classes was good, but not identifying me was good too, my recognition became personal between me and the teachers. I acknowledge that I am still a student. After these classes on literature and writing, I will have other problems. Maybe recognition in class was not a healthy thing, and I feel that, and my teachers probably know that."

"So this term paper on psychic surgery, how will the teacher read it in class?" he asked.

I felt a little embarrassed.

I apologized.

"I'm sorry, but it will never be read in class. I was supposed to graduate last year. My BS Biology was a four-year degree, and the term paper was supposed to be a group effort on that fourth year. I was taking my writing seriously, but my group mates last year, they were also my friends—we seemed to be having too much fun. Being all science majors, and most of us about to graduate, the teacher said we didn't have to concentrate on her English class too much, because we were already loaded with science subjects. She said she understood."

He asked, "So you failed and had to redo it?"

I replied, "No, their procrastination got on my nerves. I was taking my English class more seriously than they, so I deliberately got mad, stopped talking to them, and took the problem to the teacher. I told the teacher to give me an incomplete grade, I wanted out of my group, and I wanted to make my own individual term paper. I probably should not had gotten mad at my friends."

I continued, "She said 'Yes.' She gave me a grade of 'Incomplete' which gave me one additional year's time to complete it. I actually concentrated on my science courses and these last few weeks that I have been spending here with you, is actually towards the one-year deadline. I'm sorry, but your message might not be heard through my term paper."

He said "Right, but you're still missing something."

"What?" I asked.

He said, "You mentioned that you are doing all this writing to train yourself to be a writer. So that means you will eventually write about this, in a bigger and better way."

I agreed, "I had actually been thinking, a good book title would be *Psychic Philippines,* which will have different chapters on different psychic or unexplainable things and events in the Philippines. This book will take some time. But psychic surgery will be a major part of it."

"How do you hope to get your chapters written?" he asked.

"Through interviews like this," I answered.

"You are still missing something then," he smiled.

I smiled back. "What?"

"You want to go through the process of interviewing people? You remember how you got to interview me?" he asked.

"Yes? I asked to interview you, but you came to me first," I said.

"Right," he said.

"Well, my background is science, despite the overstaying and bad grades. So I think it would be good to approach all this from a scientific standpoint," I said.

He said, "Right, but what I'm saying is that if you can do psychic surgery yourself, there would be no need to interview other people. You would really lose no time interviewing by just writing about your own insights and experiences."

"You're scaring me. What you said reminds me of one of your followers. The one who is blind," I said.

"What about him?" he asked.

I continued, "Well, he has also told me that you've made other blind people see by getting rid of cataracts, and stuff like that. You and he are just a few feet away from each other every weekend. He comes here, all the time. He has told me that he believes that he will be able to see again, if you treat him. It's just a matter of him requesting you for it."

"Right, I'm willing to go through the process of making him

see, it will need several healing sessions. There are no guarantees, but he will not even begin to do it," he said.

"Yeah, he told me that, and I asked him, 'Are you scared?' He said he's used to being blind. There is no need to make him see again," I narrated.

"Yeah, I can't force another person to change if the person does not want the change," he said.

I said, "Same thing. I have heard what you preach or say to the group, I have documented what you have told me, and I have felt the goodness in the group, but I personally don't want to become a psychic surgeon."

"I have something to tell you about the power of words," he said.

"What?" I asked.

"Once you have heard the words, you will never forget them," he said.

"What do you mean?" I asked.

He continued, "You already know the principles I used to effect psychic surgery."

"Yeah?"

"It will just be a matter of time before all this sinks in, and you may just become one, a healer of sorts, if not a psychic surgeon, then something else, whether you like it or not."

I laughed. "You're scaring me, right? You're just joking?"

He laughed. "I can't really say I'm joking because what if one of these days, or years, it comes true? Will you still be laughing then?"

"No."

"You said you have plans to write in the future?" he asked.

I answered, "I think I'll become a writer and an artist. I'm still trying to figure myself out, you know, my future."

"Well, while you're trying to figure that out, then you might also try to figure out how psychic surgery will come into the picture, because it will," he said.

"I'm sure it will through my writing. I really don't think I can do psychic surgery," I said, smiling. "Like my term paper. I'll say what you said, and then I'll let the readers decide what is useful to them."

The psychic surgeon opened the Bible, once again, and read a passage in Matthew.

He said, "Christ said, 'Come unto me, all ye that labour and are heavy laden, and I will give you rest. Take my yoke upon you, and learn of me; for I am meek and lowly in heart: and ye shall find rest unto your souls. For my yoke is easy, and my burden is light."

Then he said, "Do you know what this means? This means that you can begin the process of healing other people."

I was a little puzzled. "I don't get it," I said.

"This means that Christ does not guarantee complete healing. It could happen but the emphasis is to lighten the burden of those who suffer.

"Your mere presence with hope and a good heart is a good starting point. If you are in that state of mind, then you can slowly proceed to healing other people.

"Sometimes it will happen, and sometimes it will not. But you keep training your mind to connect with people and with God, and you will eventually get it. Something will happen," he said.

"You think so?" I asked.

He answered, "I know so. You're not the only person I've told this to, and you will not be the last. Other people have learned to do what I can do. So in a way, I just keep saying what I say and preaching what I preach, and people will eventually get it."

I said, "Well, if you are saying that, then I should know more than my present knowledge, which means you have to keep teaching me."

"Well, first of all, I have already given you a lot of information. But there is something basic that you haven't even done yet," he said.

"What?"

He explained, "You have connected with me, but you have to connect directly with God. Then again, even when you say you have connected with God, there's something I'm sure you haven't done yet in your entire life."

I smiled. "What?" I asked.

"You have yet to read and study the Bible. That is where a lot of the lessons are," he said.

I agreed. "You're right. I call myself Christian and I haven't even read the Bible, but people read the Bible and haven't even begun to become psychic surgeons."

He said, "The problem with a lot of people is that they have it easy. Reading the Bible is not a requirement to go to heaven. But you must understand where I'm coming from. I myself witnessed psychic surgery before I became one. When I started listening to what the psychic surgeon before me was saying all the while, I also started thinking for myself."

He continued, "These people who are part of my group, they follow me, I talk or make a speech or give a sermon every week. They come to listen. They apply it to their lives, but they apply what I have to say to their lives as listeners, not as doers. Their mindsets are acceptable. They and you are under no pressure to change perspectives. Maybe someday, they will change their viewpoints and listen to become healers themselves."

"They are limiting themselves?" I asked.

"Well, not them, all of us are," he said.

I asked, "What do you mean?"

"All of us are limiting our own selves to a degree. Take myself for example. I have chosen to serve this way. Look at my house, I am not rich. My daughter and other kids in the neighborhood all go to public school. I remain to be a public servant in my day job. I don't write.

"You are young, you must go beyond and try to reach more. When I said that we can all tap into God, who is all-knowing, all-seeing and all-powerful, then there is much to tap into. I'm really just tapping into the healing part of God. You must find other ways to tap into God," he said.

I smiled. Then I said, "I don't understand all this yet, see, my focus is to finish a term paper."

"Right. I'm telling you all this, and you are listening and hearing, but you are still not seeing any bigger potential," he said.

I corrected him. "No, I see a bigger potential, but the task seems to be daunting."

He agreed, "Right, you will slowly ease into all this in a smoother way. It will take time."

"What else should I know?" I asked.

"Well, I've told you, you still have to read the Bible, both the Old and the New Testaments," he said.

"Okay, I will."

❧

"Here is another thought. You are a smart, educated person, I'm sure you will understand this one," he said, smiling.

"What?"

"How many books have you gone through in going to college?" he asked.

"A lot?" I said.

"How many have you gone through from the first book you've ever opened in your life?" he asked again.

"Hundreds?" I answered.

"Right. You should continue to read. You should continue to learn," he said.

I asked, "What do you mean?"

He said, "Here's a thought. There is an Old Testament, and a New Testament. No one really said the New Testament is the Last Testament. Doesn't it naturally say that there must be a Third Testament?"

"You mean it's already been written? When is the volume coming out? Don't tell me it's my term paper," I joked, then laughed a little.

"Yeah it's funny, but the Old Testament is a collection of writings. They really just put everything together for the convenience of us to read them in book form," he said.

"Right, I agree," I said.

He continued, "Then there's the New Testament which is also a collection of writings, but this time they made it convenient by saying everything in the New Testament is about Christ.

"Then there's probably a third testament that is in the works, about what happened after Christ.

"So here's my theory. Everyone is writing. Everyone is making his or her own point known nowadays. Who is to say who is correct?" he asked.

I answered, "Well, only time will tell."

"You know how the churches attempt to control its followers? By making rules and all that?" he asked.

I answered, "Well, they are there for everyone to follow in a more uniform way, that's what I think. Kind of like going to school. In school, you are given the same textbooks, and you sometimes have to wear the same uniform."

He said, "Right, but you really don't give the schoolchildren much leeway. They have to show up on time or they're late, and everyone has lunch at the same time.

"I think that when you get smarter, or when you are out of school, you have all the time to yourself, and all the time to discover God on your own, without the need for textbooks or a set schedule. You are allowed to read more and accept things on your own.

"All these books and stories and facts, and maybe even fiction. They all get printed or photographed or documented on film. This is just like the documentation which led to the Old and the New Testaments. What I'm saying is that the third testament could be all the books, and even term papers, that had been written, are being written, and will be written in future," he said.

I said, "I don't think all this will fit in a book. In speedreading class the teacher said something about the importance of speed-reading."

"What?" he asked.

"That there are thousands of titles being printed every week in the entire world, and increasing," I said. "Those are just books, not including magazines and newspapers."

"That's exactly what I'm saying. Because of our present technology, everything that is being written will probably survive. That is the Third Testament of the Bible. Everything that is written.

"What I'm saying is that your term paper is probably just as important, whether your teacher keeps it in the drawer or puts it in the library. It is as important as the single word that I told you earlier, and it is as important as when a child tells his or her parents 'I love you,' and writes it on a homemade greeting card," he said.

I asked. "What about the bad things?"

He answered, "Everything said and written are important. They all have impact. Even lies and speculations. So when the right time comes, people will make a Third Testament that will be more convenient to carry. But for now, everything is part of the making of the Third Testament. Just an idea.

☙

"If you say or write something hateful, there is impact there as well. This is my theory. There is the battle between Good and Evil. But God said, I am the Alpha and the Omega. Everything came from God and God will absorb everything in the end. Everything that is bad will be absorbed by God anyway."

I asked, "What do you mean? Are you saying that bad people will go to heaven as well?"

He replied, "Heaven and hell could be a state of mind.

"When you do something bad, then you die, there is something you have disturbed so that when God comes to you, joining back with God will hurt you a lot. Imagine getting hurt by a knife, that's a certain kind of hurt that you can imagine.

"If you can tolerate that, the hurt you will feel when God comes after you, will be much worse. That will be hell. But if you eventually get back to God, after being a good person, there is no hurt, which equates to heaven," he said.

I said, "That sounds like a good concept."

He smiled. "It works for me," he said.

※

I changed the topic. "Let's go back to psychic surgery. How can I do it assuming I get the urge to?"

"It takes time. Start psychic healing before you get to psychic surgery. Psychic surgery will happen eventually in time," he said.

I laughed. "You mean I can do all this by tomorrow?"

He replied, "No, you need to remember all that I have told you, plus spend time to read and analyze the Bible, and analyze it from a perspective of becoming a healer.

"Then you must do something else that I did, which is also crucial."

"What?" I asked.

He said, "You must spend time alone. You've heard of the saints, right?"

"There were points in their lives when they spent time alone. During that time they were able to get in touch with God and other holy beings. You must spend time alone with God," he said.

I added, "Like in a religious retreat."

He said, "More than a retreat. Retreats have set times to wake up, pray, eat, and sleep. It still follows a formula."

I asked, "What do you mean?"

He explained, "In the Bible, you will notice that the main characters spent time alone. Only then did more revelations come to them.

"There is the magic number, 40 days and 40 nights. If you can take time off to spend alone with God for 40 days and 40 nights, more or less, maybe some form of enlightenment will come to you.

"Having spent time to connect with a higher being is not just relegated to the saints. And even then, you should remind yourself that saints were ordinary people who spent time to be with God before they were declared saints. This means that ordinary people can be able to perform extraordinary things.

"A doctor for example spends time in medical school to become a doctor. That is that person's focus. If your focus is psychic healing or psychic surgery, then you follow the steps to do that. If you want to become an artist, then you follow steps to become an artist.

"If you want to become a *famous* artist, then you follow the steps to become a *famous* artist, not just be an artist. Or author, or baker. But everyone spends the time, and if you want to heal like Christ, then you should follow His teachings from a healer's perspective, and even He was not exempt from spending 40 days and nights alone, before He set out to do His mission," he said.

"So forty days and forty nights would be the way to go?" I said jokingly.

"No, I think the Bible just uses forty days and nights for convenience. What I mean to say is that you need to spend a great amount of time with God," he explained.

I said, "Hmm, it makes sense," I paused.

"I have to make a confession," I said.

"What?" he asked.

"I have been having doubts with going to medical school. I was thinking it will take time to do it," I said.

"How long?"

I answered, "About four to six more years. That's why I decided not to become one anymore. So I decided to write about psychic surgery to see if there is another way to tackle the medical field, or healing, aside from the fact that I just might have a substantial term paper project. Like killing two birds with one stone."

"What did you discover?" he asked.

I laughed a little. "That psychic surgery also takes time. And it is worse. It's scarier than medicine. There is no set formula. There are no schools. The best I can do is to write about it. Medical school also takes time.

"After coming to you, I am left with the same question."

"Which is?" he asked.

I continued, "What is my mission. What does God want me to do with my life. What you are saying, if God is the first and the last, then I have everything right here to do something with my life as my choice, and still succeed. Or not succeed."

"What is success to you?" he asked.

"Success to me is to be productive enough that God becomes happy with my own endeavors," I said.

He said, "That means you can always go back to medical school."

I said, "No, I don't think medical school is for me anymore. I'll do something else."

He asked, "Do you know that you're actually increasing your challenges?"

"What do you mean?" I asked.

He said, "Look around here. When I became a healer, I realized that there are other things that go with it."

"What?"

He explained, "A medical doctor can charge for his services. I cannot charge for my services. I have observed that charging for healing services dissipates the energy. The sick who come to me are poor. They have no money to spare. I cannot charge them anything. I can become the best psychic healer or psychic surgeon in town, and I will still be poor."

I laughed again. "Yeah, it has dawned on me that if I follow your teachings, I just might also become poor by choice. Then again, if I write about it, then I'll become a bestselling author," I joked.

He said, "Like I said, you're a smart person, you will figure all this out."

I added, "At the end of the day, I should just be happy with other people's gratitude and nothing more."

He laughed. "Haha, you must remember something else."

"What?" I asked.

"You remember the story about the lepers. Christ healed them, and only one came back to thank him."

"Oh okay. Don't expect thanks either." I laughed.

"When people come to me, their goal is to get healed. When they get healed, their goal is reached. If these people are poor, they tend to have other pressing matters, or they might also just tend to be less educated.

"These people will come to me, hoping for a cure, with no money. Some would bring gifts of food, or something else. But the majority, they do not have money. Some cannot even afford an extra jeepney fare or bus fare to come back to thank me. Some also have low self-image, they would not want to bring attention to themselves as well. When their goals are met, they do not reappear," he said.

I added, "Then there are people who might be scared by all this. To be honest with you, even as I write about psychic surgery, I'm also scared by the concept myself. Now you're also telling me that I just might be able to do it as well. That scares me even more."

He agreed, "Right, so chances are, you yourself will not come back for a while."

"Well I would not really say that," I said.

He laughed, then he said, "There are many ways of coming back.

"You don't have to be back in my presence. You can come back by having a closer relationship with God, while thinking about psychic surgery. That's just an example."

I said, "In a way, I will resolve you concept of coming back. Coming back is like giving back. To the idea. Our connection will be my submission of the paper to my teacher.

"If and when I tell someone else about all this, in the future, that will also be my way of connection or resolution. The thing about me is, I too have my problems and what bugs my mind. I'm graduating and I don't know what to do, with my entire life ahead of me."

"Right. So it's not like you would be back in the shadows like the patients I treat who don't even come back to thank me."

"No, not really," I said.

He added, "But I have accepted it as part of my outreach. That I will remain poor, I will not charge, and I will not expect for people to come back to thank me."

I asked, "And when I go on with my life, you will not expect me to come back? Does that make me a bad person?"

"No, you must remember, the goal here is not to come back to me. The goal is to connect back to God, regardless of whether you become a psychic surgeon or not. I do it and you should do it, and everyone else should do it, but there is something else."

"What?" I asked.

"When you write, you may not be a healer yourself, but your writing will serve to help others to connect to God," he said. "You remember what you said earlier about your work being read by the teacher without having to identify you?"

"What about it?" I asked.

"In school, you were praised without being identified," he said.

"Yeah?"

"There will come a time when you will find the need to be identified without being praised."

CHAPTER 38

THE LAST SUPPER

I remember going to the psychic surgeon's home for more than a month, on Sundays, maybe for six or seven Sundays.

It was many years ago, and I remember telling myself I had to stop going there to finish the term paper anyway, just in time to get a grade by the deadline for that last semester.

I actually successfully worked on the term paper on the weekdays.

Theoretically, all grades needed for graduation should be handed in by all the instructors by a certain date. It was important to make it on schedule, particularly for students like myself who had delinquent grades that might still be salvaged, in order to qualify for graduation, and to qualify to be in the graduation ceremony.

In my school, the University of the Philippines, there are two major semesters in a year, and then there is a third, more concentrated, but shorter, summer semester. Graduation dates are decided by the completion of all courses by the second semester, prior to summer. If a student completes by the summer semester, the graduation date is carried to the next year.

Since I had already overstayed by a couple of semesters, a year, my records would show a graduation date of five years after my entry into college. If I delayed on this one last piece of requirement, and my instructor submitted my grade around the a later date towards or within the summer semester, it would show on the transcript, and it would appear, that I spent six years in the university. Shameful, even by my lax standards.

I met the graduation date, when I was able to submit the term paper on time, and the teacher submitted that last passing grade on time as well.

In reality, I did not march. I thought it was embarrassing for me to do so because I had overstayed by a year. My school friends and classmates, from the batch of students I went with when I entered college, were already finishing their first year of medical school. Well, I made no plans of going to medical school anyway.

It just made no sense for me to feel as if I finished something, when I was actually searching for more meaning in my life. I felt I was lost. My graduation did not make me feel like I accomplished anything at all.

I thought that if I marched, it would feel like grandpa graduating with the kids. However, I was actually the same age, if not still younger, than some of those "kids," because I got into the university from a school which accepted me prematurely, and then accelerated me some more when I made the grade that allowed me to move from sixth grade to freshman high school without going through seventh grade.

Still, I was in search for meaning. I was still confused. Graduation seemed like I reached a pinnacle of success or some type of mental stability. Not with my type of thinking, no, I didn't think so.

Not to mention the mind-shattering, unscientific discovery of psychic surgery that I had been preoccupied with the past few months.

I thanked the psychic surgeon for all the information and time he had given me, and told him, yes, it might be a while before I saw him again, but only because I needed time to compose and finalize my English project.

I said I learned a lot from him, not mentioning that I was wrestling with the idea that what he did was suddenly a possibility in this world.

After my four or five years of scientific study in the field of Biology, here was this man who served the community free of charge, and did impossible feats that was contradictory to current scientific tenets—without the need for school.

Here was someone who gave me more meaning, but who also confused me even more.

❧

I felt I wanted to help a little or at least hang out with the group some more, but I also felt I did not want to be entangled in what I thought was a cult. I also thought I was at a very impressionable stage in my life. I was not just in a searching for meaning mode, but I was also shocked by all that I had seen in the past month or so. I needed time away from the group.

Mentally, retreat and regroup.

❧

I remember the first week when I made a promise to come back, and I asked if I could bring something. He said some cotton swabs would be nice. On the next visit, I brought a big roll of medical grade cotton, which I bought from the local drugstore chain.

That cotton was relatively expensive. I could have bought the other smaller-sized rolls.

The healer pinched from the cotton many times, and his hand as usual disappeared inside each patient. He used the cotton to blot some blood.

He placed bunches of cotton inside the patients, waved his hand to seal their wounds, leaving cotton inside the patients' bodies!

He gave instructions for the patients to come back next week so he can take the cotton out.

Each week, each biggest bundle of cotton I donated got used up! I thought there was no way I could possibly afford to do this every week. I started thinking, perhaps if he got less, he'd try to make do with that lesser amount.

I could not believe cotton could be "abused" that way. The

rolls of cotton my mother had in her medical supply each always lasted for years! I was fault-finding!

The thing was, after my Bachelor of Science in Biology, four years of academic pursuit, plus one extra overstayed year, five years total, I knew I will really flip out if I discovered then that I could do psychic surgery. I did not want to instinctively look for blood clots and get my fingers in any gaping, psychically produced wound on strangers.

※

This thought helped me to leave the Philippines. Well, maybe not really, or maybe this weight had a factor of one to five percent. How would I know for sure? I was confused in so many levels.

My joke to myself was to just ask God to give me the gift of levitation. It's a safer compromise. Now you understand, that after seeing a psychic surgeon work, I believed that I could succeed in asking God to grant me levitating abilities. Nothing was impossible with God anyway.

And even before I got the levitation deal, getting my artwork to sell for $2.4 million dollars each sounded even more realistic. More compromise.

Either way, even if God did not allow me to levitate or sell my works for $2.4 million, that's okay. Just don't make me into a psychic surgeon. The fact that the psychic surgeon said anyone can do psychic surgery, especially myself, really didn't help me.

※

Something really flipped me out the last time I went to the psychic surgeon's home. This happened in late April of that year.

I had already fulfilled the requirements of my English class. My term paper was finished, and I got a grade of A.

Two weeks before I was scheduled to leave the country for the United States, I was at the psychic surgeon's home, and with the group. They reminded me, "Val, make sure that you are here next week."

I asked why. They said that it was their anniversary, and there would be food and an election of officers.

The following week, I showed up. I was wearing my usual jeans and a shirt. The men and women were dressed better than usual. I asked where the patients were, and they said there was only going to be an election of officers and the party.

Normal stuff.

The food was humbling, because they served Filipino noodles called *pancit* ("pan-SEET"), but they "watered it down" by putting in a lot more noodles, the cheapest, bulkiest ingredient in the food, than what the spices, meat, and vegetables were able to flavor. They offered me soda, but there was only one "family-sized" bottle around, so I just had a little, and then water sufficed.

After eating, there was the election of officers, from the membership. I did not recognize most of them—they did not really go there on a regular basis. Most of them were older. The election was more for organizational purposes, it seemed. The psychic surgeon, being the founder, and only psychic surgeon in the group, remained as the main leader.

After the election, the psychic surgeon and the newly elected officers gathered around a round table with only one chair. A lady sat down on the chair, while the rest stood up. The other members, who were not officers, sat elsewhere. I was taking pictures earlier, so I was about 15 to 20 feet away from the round table. I stopped taking pictures when the atmosphere became a little more serious.

The room became quiet.

The seated lady placed her fingertips except her thumbs on a Bible placed crosswise in front of her, on the table. She closed her eyes and relaxed. Then she started to swing and rotate the Bible rhythmically, back and forth, like tracing a ribbon, you know—the left side went up, while the right side went down, then the left side went down, while the right side went up, the axis of rotation was at the center of the Bible. Back and forth, to and fro, and then she raised her head, smiled, and opened her eyes. Her strange finger play did not stop nor slow down.

She faced each one of the elected officers standing before her. Starting with the person to her left, she said in Filipino, "You, whom I love, you must do this and this and this." She gave a few sentences of pointers.

Then she faced the next person, and gave pointers again, starting with the same phrase, "You, whom I love."

"Ikaw aking iniibig,..." or "You whom I love," that phrase, in Filipino, is never really used at all, at least not in my generation.

The psychic surgeon stood in the middle of the group, so he was directly in front of her. She gave him pointers as well and proceeded to the rest of the group on the right.

She did all this in a trance, while rhythmically moving the Bible, facing all ten to twelve of them standing around that round table, from left to right. When she finished with the last person to her right, I thought she was done.

She paused and was quiet for a longer time. She stopped moving the Bible.

I was not in any kind of spotlight; I was just being silent and witnessing the event, just like everyone else. I was standing in a darker corner about 15 feet away.

Her head slowly moved and turned to me! It took me a while to realize that she was staring straight at me with unblinking eyes.

Then she spoke.

"There is someone here who is very special. He is new. He is with us only for a short time. He will leave and be gone for a very, very long time.

"You, whom I love, you will not come back to us, because your mission will take you to many other places. It will be a very long journey, and you will face a lot of problems and trials.

"You will know your mission and you will succeed. Whatever it is that you will have set yourself out to do, it is your correct path. Do it because it is the mission you and God have agreed upon. It will take years before you will see results from your mission."

She said more things to me, and I noticed that my message took longer than the ones gathered around her. I don't remember her eyes blinking. I was the only one she gave a message to who was not part of the circle of people standing by her.

After she was done talking, she turned and faced the circle again. She bowed a little, and identified the voice that was speaking through her. She mentioned a name of a saint. Then she closed her eyes, bowed her head some more, her shoulders relaxed, and with a sigh, she woke up from the trance and began to talk and act normally again.

Assuming that someone else was speaking through the lady, and all this was really true as they believed it to be, I had actually witnessed channelling even before I knew the term nor understood what it was.

I heard of the words channelling and new age only when I got into the United States and after that incident.

I had the idea to write a book then, which I wanted to call "Psychic Philippines," to feature age-old unexplainable practices and phenomena that happened in everyday Philippines. I thought, the experience with the psychic surgeon would be a chapter or two.

The world was ready for my discoveries!

But I was not.

Many reasons made me leave the Philippines, some were good and some, bad. My encounter with psychic surgery, which contradicted years of scientific study, was a factor.

This was the scary reason for my leaving. If I had stayed some more in the Philippines, I would probably had continued with my Psychic Philippines book idea, but that would had required me to go to different parts of the country. I would have had a novel, commercial idea, but a scary one, too.

I would probably had continued being with the psychic surgeon's group, but knowing myself, I would had left later on.

Displacing myself necessitated me to think of other pressing matters. The homesickness and culture shock became welcome conveniences. Later on, there was rent, a job, and my masters degree at a university in Chicago. Then art and writing.

Well, needless to say, I was really so much spooked that night. I remember not even asking anyone why I was given special attention.

I tried to act normal. I was sad.

She told the truth, that I would leave. I talked to them that night, looking into the eyes of those nice people, including the blind guy, the follower who was also more or less my age, knowing full well that night was to be my last with them.

It was nighttime. I went home using public transportation twice, as usual. I sat next to the drivers, my favorite familiar place in jeepneys.

I left the place in a dazed and confused state. I never went back.

In just a few days, I was out of the country. I never went back.

CHAPTER 39

Alien Abduction

This was a trip I described earlier. After that last visit I had with the psychic surgery group, I was on a plane bound for Chicago. In less than a week.

This was when I closed my eyes and dedicated my entire life to God as one single prayer. I had not ended the prayer.

As I write this, almost 30 years later after graduating with a Bachelors Degree in Biology and after my time with the psychic surgeon, I was quite uncertain about my future. I felt that my challenges will be greater than normal, because I thought I will be guided and I had a feeling I would not be a very practical person.

Something happened to me during this trip.

I stayed with Aunt Li for a few months. I did my visualization exercises with her. I said that in an earlier chapter as well.

Then I came back to Chicago, to stay with Mama's younger brother, Uncle Nimitz.

I was in the guest bedroom, where I slept as I normally did.

One night, I slept somewhat differently. I felt high. I remember comparing my groggy state to having taken strong, cold medication.

With a sudden jerk, as if I were suddenly dropped back on my bed, I awoke, startled. This sudden jerk alone was puzzling enough, but what I did next was even more mystifying. It was as if I knew I had to do it as soon as possible, but it was as if I had forgotten why I had to do it.

I suddenly felt the need to really wake up, compose myself, get up, stand on the side of the bed, take my shirt off and look for something on my body. I felt that there was something on my body, but I can't seem to remember where it was and what it was.

I finally saw what I thought I needed to look for.

Right smack in the middle of my front, just below my sternum, where my diaphragm begins, was a round, red to purplish scoop mark that seemed to already be healing. I never had it the night before.

A few weeks later, the mark not only continued to remain, and continued to be red in color, but it formed a keloid. It was like a bump just larger than a pimple that had a central puncture scar.

☙

I had a benign sebaceous cyst on my left buttock that had to be taken out about a week after I started seeing the psychic surgeon. The surgery left a 2-inch elongated scar which became keloid and bumpy. Uncle Nick injected steroid into it a few times to flatten the bump. I also learned through the years that keloid skin flattens if you kept scratching it. The scar on my butt stayed but the keloid bump flattened.

☙

I also scratched this keloid scoop mark every once in a while, through the years. The dark reddish spot remains, but the bump had flattened.

☙

I thought this was an isolated incident. The last strange sleep that woke me up, startled and high. About 8 years later and living elsewhere, the sensation of being high came back.

I was asleep, but while sleeping, it seemed as if I became conscious that I was sleeping. Then I realized that the same sensation of being high was back.

I jerked again, as if I was once again lifted and dropped on the bed, and suddenly woke up.

"Oh no, it's happened again," I told myself. I suddenly stood up and turned the light on. This time, I searched my legs first.

I saw a red scoop mark again. It was bumpy when I pressed it in. I knew it would become keloid through the years. This time it was near my right knee, on the right side and about two inches below the level of the knee.

I still have both marks today. I never bothered to keep scratching on the second one. It's still bumpy. Once in a while, it itched.

༄

Years after that, I noticed that I always had a tiny bump behind either my left or right ear. Then I developed a permanent tinier one behind my left ear, but it can't be a pimple since it never went away. I can feel it. It used to irritate me, but years later I learned to stop caring to find out about it.

༄

I wonder if I may have been tagged.

༄

When Borders Bookstore was still open downtown, when I still lived downtown, I used to go to the Paranormal / UFO section just to check out the titles.

I had been going to the annual publishers convention and through the years I came to know David Hatcher Childress, an author-publisher of strange archeology-based books. I used to pass by his exhibition booth daily during the show. On the last day, towards closing time, he used to give me all the books I cared to take from his display so he didn't have to bother with them, because he was exhausted and ready to just go home, just like all of us.

On one trip to the convention, I gave him a pen that blinked colored lights. It reminded me of UFOs, so I made sure I gave him one. He was going to give me his displayed books anyway.

I got into just looking at David's books at Borders to remind me of the magical book convention, and then check out what else was on the shelves.

One day at Borders, I was relaxing and familiarizing myself

with the Paranormal / UFO section, when a man stood next to me to check out the same section. He too seemed to be studying the section.

I said hello, and we started to talk.

He said he was a doctor, but he was into UFOs.

I jokingly asked him if he wanted to see my marks, because I believe I may had been abducted by aliens in my sleep.

I lifted up my shirt, showed him the mark on my abdomen, and then lifted my right pants leg to show him the other one by my knee.

He reached for the shelf and pulled out a book about alien implants from the shelf. It was *Casebook: Alien Implants (Whitley Strieber's Hidden Agendas)* by Roger Leir and Whitley Strieber. He said I should check it out.

I said thanks for the tip.

I bought the book and went home.

ಎ

There's something else too. I used to get a lot of nosebleeds. Between the '80s and '90s, I got between 2 to 7 nosebleeds each week. I figured it must be the dry air, especially during winter.

When I lived with my uncle around the first time I felt I may have been "taken," I never told him anything. I didn't want him to worry and have me sent to the Philippines. He might think I was sick and needed medical attention. I didn't have insurance here. I also did not want anyone else to worry about this. These incidents worked against my future.

When I lived alone in the '90s, I took my nosebleeds for granted, but they became more frequent.

Over this last decade and a half, I stopped getting nosebleeds, but I always had a scab healing inside my right nostril.

ಎ

The scab disappeared just this year, in 2013. My two red

marks and whatever is behind my left ear remain.

⁂

Well, here's how I debunk this one. I got numerous ECGs and CBCs through the years. CBC stands for Complete Blood Count—a complete profile of what is in the blood. I started participating in medical studies because of the ECGs and CBCs. Always normal. There's nothing wrong with me.

Chapter 40

Shadows & The Dream

I moved to downtown Chicago in 1998 to get nearer the hotels, timed with the first ever inclusion of my massage ads in the yellow pages. I made money from massage based on the ads I had in the yellow pages. My stories of becoming a masseur is in the other memoir, **Leadership Rubs: 1-Hour Mentors.**

In 2001, I was amazed at how I got from struggling and poor to impoverished and totally hopeless in the blink of an eye.

I thought the two competing yellow page companies were reliable. I had my apartment lease and obviously needed to make the rent and other expenses every month. 2001 was when the leading yellow page phone book failed to include my massage ad. February was the month when the new book came out. Tons of copies were at my apartment building's walkway where the shipping room was. I opened one, looked for my ad, and it was not there! I felt my blood rise and fill my head. Common sense told me that as the phone books got delivered to the apartment buildings, all the hotels had also efficiently placed the new ones in all their rooms.

I quickly placed local ads in the weeklies. This was the year when I decided to place ads in all the competing yellow page companies. The competing phone book was smaller and not used by all the hotels. It came out toward the end of the year.

Since when I moved in 1998, I was not making enough money to buy a bed. I used a cheap inflatable bed, which in time had tiny holes in it. I inflated it at night, but by morning it had deflated and I ended up waking on the hard carpeted floor.

I lived in a small studio apartment. I did not bother getting a remote phone because they too were expensive, and I assumed that they would stop working when dropped. What I did was connect two old 25-foot telephone wires so I was able to walk all over the tiny place while still on the phone.

I also did not want to have a regular bed. I wanted a loft bed I saw at Ikea. I had massage clients who came to my place. I never liked people sitting on the edge of my beds in the past. If I had a regular bed in the same room as my clients, they might end up sitting on the bed or worse, wanting to do something else besides massage. The loft bed I saw was about 6 feet above the ground, and I can use the space under the bed for a computer table or storage. I was able to save up for this the next year.

My home phone, which had caller I.D., was always next to me, just in case I got a massage call. When I slept, I had it next to me, with the 50-foot wire collected under the phone in an unruly fashion. When I went to the hotels to do massage, I forwarded my calls to my cellphone. This was the time when cellphone rates were still high and it was more economical to maintain a home landline.

Next to the phone was my electronic clock radio, which had a large red LED display.

By the time I woke up, my inflatable bed had deflated, and my head usually had shifted over the phone wire.

☙

One fateful night, I suddenly woke up. It was still dark. I looked at the clock. It said 3:00. Weird, I thought, because it was exactly 3:00 a.m.

My next immediate observation was that the room seemed like it was just too dark. I cannot see much. It felt like I was surrounded by shadows. It felt like there were some entities that were so black they seemed to be devoid of light, in the room, standing, looking down at me lying at floor level on a deflated airbed. There was no ambient light coming from outside and through the blinds.

I got so scared, I closed my eyes. I wondered what to do next. Then I thought that if there were more than just myself in my room, I should try to talk to them and see what happens next.

I said in a loud voice, "If you can hear me, I am worried and suffering financially. I could really use some help so if you can send money my way, I would really appreciate it."

I kept my eyes closed until I fell asleep. Then I started dreaming.

The things moving in my dream was a monochromatic light brown, the background and floor were pitch black. What I was seeing was very vivid. I became aware and came to the realization that I was dreaming. I recalled that shadowy figures were in my room earlier, and so I told myself that I should just enjoy and stay in this dream as long as possible. The visitors might still be at my place.

In my dream, I saw American civilians, in office clothes running, emerging out of billowing smoke. Going into the smoke were soldiers in uniform, with guns in hand.

I heard, "Syria is attacking the United States! Syria is attacking the United States!"

As I heard people shouting that, I became aware of a few things. First I knew I was dreaming. I was happy and relieved to have obviously slept after having been visited by shadow people.

I noticed that the dream was dark. It was pitch black except for the smoke and the people. With civilians dressed the way they were, in office clothes, I wondered why it was dark that way when it should have been bright. The smoke was only about 5 feet away from me, but it was not dissipating. The workers were coming out of the smoke from 5 feet away; the soldiers from behind me were entering the smoke just 5 feet in front.

At first, I thought the dream was in sharp black and white. Shortly afterwards, I realized that the color was ashy brown. Their clothes, faces and hair did not show any colors other than light grayish brown. While the civilians and the soldiers were rushing at normal speed, the smoke behaved like it was solid and in slow motion.

I approached the cloud of smoke, wondering why it was not

dissipating normally. As I stared at it, I saw that it was made of tiny particles suspended in the air! I wasn't staring at smoke. I was staring at dust stopped in midair!

I discerned that the place was a stairwell, the emergency exit of an office building. It was daytime, but the emergency lights were probably blocked by the dust, I thought. The people were brownish gray-colored because they were covered in the dust!

The dream was over. I continued to sleep. The next thing I knew, I awoke to my phone ringing next to my head. It was morning. I was lying on the hard floor, the air bed had deflated as usual. I had moved off the airless plastic bed and my head was on top of the phone cord.

I was so exhausted from my lack of sleep, but relieved that sunlight was back in my room. I looked at the phone's caller ID, saw that it was Dori, a close friend, let the phone continue ringing, and went back to sleep.

The phone rang again. Same caller. This time I thought I probably should answer it. It was Dori at her store / art gallery. Dori was a friend who was older. She had two sons in Chicago, one of whom was my age, but Dori and I were closer friends.

We talked everyday when she was still in Chicago and owned and ran that store with mostly Filipino books, gifts and fine art by Filipino artists. We had a few common denominators. She had sponsored and curated some art shows that I was included in a few times in the past. She finished with a degree in Fine Art from the same university that I got my bachelors degree. We also used to contribute to the same free Chicago Filipino community paper.

Lately, she had been complaining about her computer. I thought she must need help with it if she had to call me twice that morning.

I answered the phone, I looked at my clock. It was morning, thank God, no more shadowy figures.

"Hello?" I pretended to be alert and fully awake.

"Turn on the TV!" she exclaimed.

"What channel?" I asked.

"Any channel." she answered.

I turned the TV on and watched. Weird. I saw a scene that was somewhat similar to my dream!

"Oh my God, I dreamt this!" I told her.

"What do you mean?" she asked.

"I was dreaming before you called!" I told her what happened to me earlier, from the 3 a.m. visitation to the dream. I told her about the dark, scary shadows and the dream of the soldiers and the dust. Weird. I had premonitions before, but this topped them all.

We exchanged ideas about what happened to me, then I thanked Dori, and told her I would call her back later. I had just woken up and needed to compose myself. I had a weird, energy-sapping night, and now this!

I put the phone down and continued to watch the television, switching channels between CBS, ABC, NBC, CNN, CNN Headline News, and CNBC.

౿

This happened on September 11, 2001. 9/11. When the planes crashed into the World Trade Center.

౿

My dream was almost accurate but not quite. In my dream, I heard the country Syria mentioned, but that was not the country involved. I also saw soldiers go into the smoke, not the New York police and firefighters. In hindsight, maybe I saw the Pentagon?

౿

Around 11 a.m., I called the Philippines and talked to Dinna. They were also watching the news. I told her of my ghostly visitors and the dream. Then I put the phone down.

The phone rang again. It was Dinna again. "Mama wants to talk to you."

I talked to my mom and recanted my story.

She said, "Do you know it must had been Tito Nick visiting you? It was just his birthday, September 10. How do you compute the half day difference between there and here?"

"Okay that's really weird. I never remember anyone's birthdays past our immediate family's," I said.

Through the years, because I was still struggling and did not want to get nostalgic, I stopped computing ages or remembering birthdays except those of my immediate family's. Kuya Jing and Amel each had kids. I did not want to get into the habit of calling the Philippines just to greet people on their birthdays. They might expect phone calls and timely gifts which I cannot afford.

Maybe Tito Nick did visit me, and I also dreamt of the disaster. Who knows. Maybe it was all coincidence.

☙

So here is what I think happened to me, if anyone will believe it.

I had never heard phone conversations nor television noises from my neighbors next door through the years that I lived where this happened. My floor and ceiling were concrete. No one stayed too long in the hallways for me to hear conversation.

I slept next to a regular phone that was connected to the wall. It's tangled 50-foot cord was under my head when I woke up. My sleep was uncomfortable. Maybe, something about the electronics, electromagnetism or the wiring made me sensitive or made me dream.

I was also in a depressed, worrisome state. Something stirs up in the mind when you are depressed.

Here is my view of my glass being half empty. My dream was wrong. I heard the wrong country and saw soldiers, not police and firefighters.

Here is my view of my glass being half full. By the end of that week, it occurred to me, I had two paranormal incidences in just one night. Not bad.

A year later, the undiagnosed depression I suspected I had was gone. My yellow page ads for massage were in place in the 2002 books. I finally bought a handset cordless phone. I put away my 50-foot cord.

When the tsunami in Asia happened, in 2004, I did not experience anything paranormal. I figured it was probably because I was no longer depressed.

Whoever reads this, if you want to experiment, Connect your home landline to a fifty-foot telephone cord and sleep on it for a few nights. See if vivid, seemingly prophetic dreams come to you.

Chapter 41

Snakes in the Woods

My phone rang once in a while, and it would be Papa.

"Hello, Val, *anak!*" was Papa's usual greeting, even when he left messages in the voice mail.

I always answer with "Hi, Pa!"

Or "Hi Ma!"; "Hi Dinna!"; "Hi Amel!"; "Hi K'Jing!"

"K'Jing" or "kuh-JING" is how we siblings usually pronounce "Kuya Jing" in a fast way. Another version, pronounced, "Kooy Jing," is our less popular fast pronunciation. My sisters cannot do that with my name. They usually pronounce mine the right way, "Kuya Val." The fastest way would be "KOOY Val." The "V" did not allow for not mentioning the "Y."

Mama would say "Hi, Val!" but I don't remember hearing Papa say "hi." He always used "hello," followed by my name, and then by *anak*, which in Filipino means "child," a shortened way of saying "my child."

I used to wonder if he adopted me, until I noticed that I started looking a little like him and other relatives. My brother had the face of my mom when she was about four years old, so I was sure he was not adopted.

☙

In 2011, Papa and I were on the phone, talking for hours, small talk, thanks to a Magic Jack. His phone was connected via the internet, thanks to the contraption, and my cellphone had unlimited talk.

He mentioned that one of the family's trusted farm help from decades ago came to Manila and visited him. The man had an interesting story, he said, and now I'm sharing it with you.

It was summer break and there was this young man who had just graduated from college in Manila. His parents, who sent him to school, were farmers who lived on Lubang Island.

Right after graduation, he boarded a boat for Lubang. The boat arrived late in the afternoon. He got on a jeepney with some other passengers to take him home about a few kilometers away from the pier, which was in Tilik. I don't know which small barrio his parents lived. A jeepney is the colorful, well-decorated Filipino public transportation that seated about 16 people. Its front looks like a version of a wartime Jeep. You can go online for how it looks like.

Along the way, he asked the driver to stop. His stomach was bad and he requested for them to stop so he can poop, maybe behind some bushes. By this time, it had gotten dark.

The driver stopped and the young man rushed to the bushes and disappeared.

A few minutes later, he came up and claimed that something bit him as he did his business. It must had been a snake, he said, because he had started to feel weird.

My dad said the guy died, but he was not sure if the guy died on the way to his parents or if he was able to stay alive just in time for him to see his parents. The guy went to school, graduated, got his diploma and came back to the island, only to die, unintentionally.

☙

"Filipino" is the English or Spanish word that refers to the national language or the people from the Philippines. "Pilipino" is when it is spelled in a Filipino language book. The feminine "Filipina" and "Pilipina" refer to women. Spain gave the country it's name, "Filipinas," in honor of King Philip II of Spain, but when the U.S. took over, the spelling for the country changed to "Philippines."

The national language, Filipino, is actually the "Tagalog"

language, the language spoken in Manila, but Tagalog also refers to the region where it has been originally spoken. Hence Tagalog has a "regional" connotation, but as the accepted national language taught all over the country, the politically correct term to use is "Filipino."

Lubang Island speaks Tagalog, or Filipino. The island locals speak it with an accent. The way Filipino is spoken by the locals in Manila and on Manila-based television news compares to the way English is spoken on television news in the U.S., the General American accent, which some also call a Generalized Midwestern accent.

There is a Tagalog phrase, *"Tabi po"* ("tah-BEE pò") used by the Tagalogs where they lived. The other regions understand it, but seldom use it. "Tabi" means "to the side" or "by the side." "Po" is a term of respect to an elder with a slight hint of "please." The way it is pronounced sounds like the "u" in "uh-oh."

People say it when they need to answer the call of nature, and there's no bathroom. They "superstitiously" assume that when peeing, or pooping, in nature, that there may be unseen entities nearby. It would not hurt to say "Tabi po" just to be safe.

༒

Sometimes, we're in search of bigfoot and UFOs, we forget that there are real physical dangers out there.

There are snakes in the Philippines. Some of them are constrictors and some of the are venomous. Sometimes they find their way in dark basements or ceilings and attics.

Lubang Island has snake roadkill on the Main Road. They look like long straight logs with both ends flattened. We saw them, but we never bothered to check them out. It was just a given. Where they came from, there must be more.

By the side of the road, by the dry ditches and by the side of hills and cliffs, are burrows in the soil. People say snakes live in those holes. I had never seen anyone try to coax a snake out of those burrows, not even curious kids. I wonder what are really in those burrows.

Crabs burrow too, but theirs are towards the shore, just above the high tide sea level, or below it, so they show up during low tide.

Constrictors even end up in urbanized Manila.

When I was small, in the '70s, in Manila, I saw about 10 street kids carry a very long, dead snake that was as thick as a football and at least fifteen feet long. They were clutching it with their left arm, as they shared the weight. They were followed by even more kids. That was a rare, sensational find.

Around 1998, my dad found and killed a constrictor in the house in Manila. It fell down from the rafters, breaking a portion of the ceiling. At first, he thought it was a cat. Our house was big, he did not immediately run to the room where it happened. Luckily, he saw it slither away in a very slow manner. It was about twenty feet, and quite thick. He used a crowbar and a broom to send it to snake heaven. He told me it had probably been living in the rafters for a long time. Something that huge could not had just gone up there lately.

CHAPTER 42

THE 1940s PSYCHIC HEALER

Papa had a collapsed right lung. Actually, even his right rib cage had collapsed. Even his right nipple was sunk in.

When he used to work in an office, he went to this famous tailor in Manila, where they padded the suits and jackets they tailor-made for him, to make him look balanced and upright. In just a regular shirt, he looked like he had a bad case of scoliosis.

When we were kids, Mama teased him, calling him "'ling." Then she joked, "You can't be sure if ''ling' stands for Darling or *Kiling*."

Kiling, pronounced "kee-LING," is Filipino for "bend" or "bent."

☙

During World War II, Papa's family had to escape the Japanese. They were in Mariveles, Bataan, which was part of the famous Death March. Obviously, the Japanese were there because the Americans were there. In the thousands, which meant that Bataan was urbanized and quite progressive, but I'm sure it was still tamer than Manila back then, as it still is now. This was also the birthplace of my grandma, *Lola* Inay ("Grandma Inay," pronounced "eeh-NA-yee"). We didn't really ask if our grandparents fell in love or if the marriage was arranged. My grandpa's brother *Lolo* Indo ("Grandpa Indo") also married my grandma's half-sister, Lola Clarita. My grandpa, Lolo Jesus, and Lolo Indo brought their families to Lubang Island.

The split, from one single province, Mindoro, into two current provinces, Occidental Mindoro and Oriental Mindoro happened in 1950, after the war.

Lubang Island was not without its Japanese occupiers, but the place was more laid back, even now. When my siblings and I went there for summer vacation, especially in the '70s, we had to use candles and kerosene lamps at night. Grandpa also had some bright Coleman lanterns that had to be pumped. They shone more steadily and were as bright as halogen lamps.

Their house was in Tilik, where the pier was.

The occupation by the Japanese on Lubang Island was more low-key, but there were times when the men were lined up and threatened. The residents still saw dogfights in the sky. There were stories when bombs were dropped on Lubang Island, but they were mostly unintentional. There was no reason to drop bombs on slow, laid-back Lubang Island.

With the bombs and crashing planes came undetonated bombs. Dynamite fishing was still not outlawed then. Papa said that one time they saw a dog with something in its mouth. They stopped the dog to see what it was holding. It was a human being's penis! Papa said some residents tried dismantling bombs thinking they can use the explosives for dynamite fishing.

Lolo Jesus owned horses then.

Papa's collapsed lung was the result of him falling off a horse around a year after the war. For fear of getting punished, he did not tell his dad what happened. Papa broke a rib or two, but it must had been worse, and the right lung probably got punctured.

His condition worsened. Eventually, they had to bring him to Manila, where he was hospitalized at Quezon Institute. Quezon Institute then was a hospital with a sprawling compound where people with tuberculosis were treated.

Papa claimed that his horse panicked and threw him off when they came to a path that had what seemed to be white powder on the path. I'm sure, knowing how strict my grandparents were, he stuck to that story, whether it was accurate or not.

Kuya Jing and I also rode on Lolo Jesus' later horses when we were young in the '70s. We rode and rode and rode and rode, until

Kuya Jing's horse lost its balance. Only then did it occur to us that we should probably take the horses to the river to drink.

Papa stayed in the hospital for many months. His family then was conscious about status. Quezon Institute was famous as a tuberculosis hospital. It was embarrassing to be there.

The time came for Papa to finally be taken home to die. This was our home in Manila before it was rebuilt. They said they bought the property because of the need for Papa to be hospitalized in Manila.

☙

Here is where psychic healing came into play.

When they got home, they asked a faith healer to have a look at Papa. Lola Tesay was there too. This faith healer, a lady, came to our address, to the original house that stood then.

They said she laid her hands on him. How long her healing session took, I never found out. Papa was not totally conscious. He was dying. Lola Tesay never wanted to elaborate, because the entire situation was simply scary for her.

In a nutshell when they first talked about this to us in the '70s, I remember they said a lot of pus came out of Papa through his nipple. They said it was so bad it was green in color and smelled horribly. The faith healer kept pressing until nothing more came out. From that point on, he got better, but his ribs remained misshapen and his right lung no long functioned.

☙

On that day, after administering to Papa, the healer took a look at Lola Tesay, who then supposedly wore high prescription glasses.

The healer asked if she wanted to stop wearing glasses. Lola Tesay said yes. Supposedly, the healer used saliva on her eyes, adjusting the vision by spitting into her eye at least a couple of times as the healer asked Lola Tesay if the vision needed to improve some more.

Lola Tesay swore by this story. She never again needed to wear glasses, except decades later when she needed the mild ones for reading. Ever since I can remember, up until the last time I saw her, when she was in her 70s, I never saw her wear anything but reading glasses. She died at a nursing home when she was 90.

⁂

A few months ago, Dinna mentioned a related story. Lolo Jesus once confided in her a story he never told the rest of us.

During World War II, Lolo Jesus was lined up together with other men in the village. They were blindfolded with their hands tied behind their backs. They were made to bow down. This was in Bataan, which was part of the famous Death March, the reason they had to escape to Lubang.

One by one, the blindfolded men were beheaded. Lolo Jesus was the last in the line of victims for that day's war atrocity.

He prayed silently, in his heart and mind. "Saint Michael the Archangel, save me."

The Japanese leader who gave the command told the soldier with the sword to stop.

The leader approached Lolo Jesus. He gave Lolo Jesus a massage on the shoulders. He personally untied my grandpa and took off his blindfold. The man told my grandpa to go home and return to his family.

Nowadays, I pray to the angels. I was born on a Tuesday, and Tuesday, according to the new age websites is assigned to the Archangel Raphael.

In my prayers, I honor all the angels, but I especially acknowledge Michael and Raphael.

CHAPTER 43

VIBRATIONAL ENTITIES

If I did not include this chapter, I would not have told you everything.

First, I will water this chapter down with a stupid nonparanormal story, followed by a more paranormal story that I cannot bring myself to believe, and then my own story, which I personally believe to be true. I'm saying "believe" because I could have been dreaming, albeit vividly, I just did not want to admit it.

※

When we kids were small, our parents raised chicken in Manila for the eggs. We had a huge garage, so Papa converted a portion into shelves of separated hens. The floors were inclined so that the eggs rolled out of the cages to the front gutter as soon as they were laid. Papa even labeled the cages with female names. Sometimes, we saw the moment when the eggs came out of the chicken butts. Our most memorable resident of that chicken condo was Candida.

As Candida laid her egg, us kids and Papa coaxed her, "Come on, Candida! You can do it! We believe in you! Yaay! Candida! Yaay!" Mama thought we made the chicken not want to lay eggs.

So we accumulated chicken feed sacks made of printed cotton. Mama had them made by the neighbor into house shorts with garter waists for myself, my brother and my sister, and small-sized pillow cases for our heads when we slept.

As small kids, we ran around, we were dirty and we stunk. What we liked to do with the pillows, we each held one all day long, from the morning and onwards and sat on them, rubbing our dirty asses on those supposedly dainty, little rectangular pillows with color prints, and at night we either had them under our heads, or we hugged them with our legs and peed into them as we slept. This was why Mama always had new pillows made on a regular basis, made from the sacks of chicken feed, but she complained to us that the cotton filling was expensive.

We had second floor windows that had wrought iron enclosures, so we can sit on the panes and not fall off. These windows overlooked the tailors. We were not even pre-school age then, but our tailoring neighbors saw myself, my brother and my sister in the chicken feed shorts, get on the window panes, pull down our chicken feed shorts, relieve ourselves, pull back up our shorts, and then take the tiny pillows they made for us and sit our dirty asses in the chicken feed shorts down on the chicken feed pillows.

Here's the big lie which we believed. Both Mama and our lady tailoring neighbor—she and her husband were both tailors—told us, on that one afternoon, and they both seconded the motions of each other, that we will develop those infected, gigantic boils with eyes in the centers on our butts and our groins, if we continued to sit on the pillows all day long and if we hugged the pillows with our legs at night.

We kids got terrified and stopped sitting on the pillows in the morning and hugging them at night with our legs.

When we got old, we figured out that it was their ingenious way of discouraging us from messing the pillows up.

❧

Around grade school, Mama's sister came to Manila for something and here's her story.

There was this old man in the village, who denounced God. He said he was not happy with God and so he had declared to give his soul to the devil. He had told that to people in the village, so it became common knowledge.

My aunt said that this man finally was at his deathbed, and on the day he died, there were his relatives and the priest who was giving him the Catholic last rites, in the bedroom with him.

As the priest prayed, loud enough for the other people in the room to hear and participate in, everyone felt the rustling and heard the sound of small invisible footsteps in the room, as if small invisible entities were scampering about.

They noticed that the bed cover and the curtains moved as if those beings were brushing up against the fabrics as they moved like small pets would, and there seemed to be a good number of them.

They felt small, invisible entities brush up against their legs, pants and skirts.

The old man died, but it was not a peaceful death. The scampering stopped when he drew his last breath. My aunt guessed that he probably saw who were picking him up, and they were not good entities.

I listened to this with fascination, but with a little incredulity. It was a good, animated story, coming from my aunt, but in retrospect, having become a writer, this story could have been a fabrication as a way for kids to become more religious. Now it sounds like an urban legend.

༄

So here's one of my "latest" stories, 2013.

I had started to "desperately" pray for my dad. I had even started praying the rosary and the Stations of the Cross when I was laying in bed. Both prayers took a long time to finish. I cannot say all this was a "sacrifice," because my heart was in it and I enjoyed doing it.

If this were a video game, I would say that my praying and devotion felt like a sort of "leveling up." I got to the point where I felt I had become more spiritual, and whatever mental or spiritual state I felt as I "ascended," had not plateaued yet.

My bed was an aluminum loft bed that was about 5 feet from the floor. It used to be higher, but I cut some inches off of the four aluminum pipes that were the legs-turned-posts. I used to have a computer table in the area under the bed. I later put a folding chair bed—a folding overnight bed as wide as a big chair and narrower than a twin bed in the area.

I must had been a nasty sinner before all this religious activity, because it did seem like there were scampering movements under my loft bed. On the other hand, it could also had been my neighbor's dog or cat, in the apartment just above me. The sound and vibrations may had bounced down to my floor before I felt it.

What I'm saying here is that I have no proof, and I never wanted proof. I never set up infrared cameras or anything, nor did I ask for whatever invisible presence to make itself or themselves known to me. I never entertained it. I just knew I was going to write about this because this might also happen to others.

I also never felt fear. I thought it was a natural occurrence.

We all talk about the belief that as we attract good, there is the bad that will complain and make its presence and dissatisfaction known. Some people believe that as we attract good luck, something else happens. At the very nonparanormal state, when someone gets a promotion at work, someone else will express an obviously intangible, but obvious negative emotion of envy.

So I heard and felt scampering a few times. Then they went away. My theory was that I got stronger spiritually. I did not acknowledge their presence, so they left.

However, within that time period as well, which was a span of about a week and a half, I was asleep again. I was sleeping and laying on my stomach, when I awoke to feel a buzzing vibration coming from within myself and permeating throughout my entire body, from my head to my toes. In my mind, it felt like it came from a good supernatural source. I was comfortable and did not panic. There was real vibration happening to me that sounded like a "zzz" from an electric shaver.

This happened two full times and two "half" times.

That event I described above was the first.

The second time it happened, I was in bed again, my entire body started to vibrate again with that familiar "zzz" buzzing noise.

This time, I was laying on my back. I had my eyes closed all the while, as usual. I knew I enjoyed this the first time, so I turned over to lie on my stomach in order for me to enjoy the vibration on my back even more.

I maneuvered myself, still with eyes closed, the vibration still happening, and I succeeded, except that after a few seconds, I began to feel that someone was touching my shoulder, attempting to forcefully turn me back over. I shrugged it off but the pull was hard enough that I had to turn over. I opened my eyes, and looked at who was doing it.

I saw what looked like a slim person, propped up, reclining next to me as well, but the entire being looked like a gray, faceless static, like the static of an old television screen on a channel that did not have a signal. The vibrating, massaging feeling was the same as the first time, and I was surprised that I trusted that seemingly gray vibrational entity. I turned over like it wanted me to do, calmly closed my eyes again, enjoyed the buzz, and fell asleep.

Days later, for a couple more times, I felt the vibration start, while I was wide awake in bed. Both happened when I was praying very intently. These next two occurrences, I attempted to see if I can control the phenomenon. I discovered that if I stopped praying and thought about something else, it stopped.

I have yet to know what these instances were all about. I wasn't imagining them, but I cannot be 100% sure what they were. I initially thought I got grounded from an adapter plug, because I slept alone on a full-sized loft bed and all my adapters were on the left side of the bed, while I slept on the right side.

I told Papa this and he also said he felt vibration when he prayed before the same Virgin Mary in the church owned by my school, while next to his brother who way back had an unknown, debilitating disease. They were getting ready to mortgage a property to send Uncle Nick to the U.S., to get diagnosed and treated. Uncle Nick was not just a doctor then. He was head of a medical school. He had connections in the medical field, and still, no one could find out what he had, why he was in pain when he peed and why he could not even stand up straight without being in pain.

So on that day with Uncle Nick in church, Papa was praying, then he felt vibration from a shoulder to his hand. He touched my uncle and confidently told my uncle that he was healed.

Papa claimed that after that prayer in church, my uncle got better. They did not have to mortgage any property after all.

I'm sure I'm not alone to have had this experience.

I'm honestly writing all this down, because I'm sure I was not the first to experience all this. Papa's experience may had been the same as mine. Maybe it's something physical that gets triggered in the brain. Someone else will come forward.

CHAPTER 44

PRAYERS

In this chapter, I am writing about my religious fanaticism, because I think this is important, in case I become a candidate for sainthood 150 years from now. I'm being funny.

I think this is important, in case you make an attempt to become an overnight healer. I must tell you that in my opinion, I "failed" being a healer. There might also be a better approach than what I did. On the other hand, I believe that my approach is valid, at least to me and God. Once again, all this is about faith.

What you can do is either try to surpass what I did, or find a better way.

☙

August and September 2013. Papa was not getting better. Being that I was in Chicago, and he was in the Philippines, there was nothing much I can do but pray.

I checked up on Papa, Mama, Dinna and Kuya Jing every once in a while. I sent them email from my phone, but I was only able to wait for them to call or message me from their phones.

I had given three Magic Jacks to my family in the Philippines. One went to Papa's home, so Papa, Mama and Dinna would be able to call me, another went to my brother Jing and the third one went to Amelia. Amel lives with her husband and kids on the island of Bohol.

The Magic Jack is a tiny little gadget which is plugged into a computer's USB port. A regular landline telephone is plugged into the Magic Jack. As long as the computer is online, a dial tone is produced.

I registered the three in Chicago, with local phone numbers, and sent the three to them. The problem was that they did not always have their computers turned on, and they only plugged their Magic Jacks in when they felt like calling me. I was at the mercy of them calling me first; I can't call them.

Papa and I used to talk for hours, thanks to the Magic Jack. If their internet connection was weak, the connection got cut off. They simply just redial.

What I was able to do was email my brother from my phone. He was able to setup his Android phone to receive emails. I simply asked him to ask Dinna to call me back.

Still, they all claimed to be busy. Dinna was the only one taking care of Papa and Mama, and Papa had cancer. I asked for daily calls, which never happened. There were times when they didn't call me for 2 weeks!

Here I was in Chicago, unable to call them, preoccupied with worry about Papa, and no updates. I knew he was getting worse, because my brother had begun to update me more regularly, from his Magic Jack, from his home, which was about 2 hours away from Manila.

The Magic Jack company came up with a phone app that did not need the device. My brother was eventually able to set it up on his phone, but it took a while for him to get the app to work on Dinna's phone. With the app, all they needed was to be where there was wi-fi.

☙

As I mentioned earlier, I got into the habit of spending more and more time praying.

I'm Catholic. I started to search for prayers online, looking for "formulaic," already written Catholic prayers that I had not yet discovered. I saw some websites and printed out some prayers. I was being cheap. For more than a month, I recited prayers from printouts.

Then I searched online for nearby Catholic stores. I discovered a gift shop located in the basement of a downtown church, St.

Peter's Catholic Church, and for a while I went there about every week, buying prayer books and prayer cards. Prayer cards are those cards that are just a little bigger than a business card. They have a picture of a saint or Christ or some other religious figure on one side and a prayer on the other side. I figured they had the choice, special prayers. I thought the thicker prayer books had a more random collection.

At the gift shop, I saw empty plastic bottles that had "Holy Water" imprinted in gold foil. I learned that anyone can bring home holy water. I just needed to buy the cheap plastic bottle, have it blessed by the priest or monk upstairs, and dip the bottle into the well just before where the pews were. I bought a bottle.

I also bought those little medals that had religious images on both the front and back. These were mostly made of aluminum. Some people believe that these medals have powers after being blessed. I don't believe this, I think they were nice to collect. They reminded me about my faith and devotion.

These things are called "sacramentals." It is believed that once these items get blessed, then they become indestructible, not physically, but religiously. Supposedly they have religious importance and that's why exorcists have sacramentals during exorcisms. On a normal basis, they are nice to have, and that belief of holiness helps the layperson.

This was how I coped with their lack of communication. I communicated with God, and communicated even more than before. I had always been religious, but, for Papa, I got seriously into praying every chance I can get!

Before September 2013, I had so many bouts of frustration with Papa, Mama and Dinna. Even Kuya Jing. By the time they called me, I ended up shouting at Papa, Mama or Dinna, for neglecting to call me, for making me worry and for what? By the time they called me, they were all cheerful and well-adjusted, Papa was dying of cancer, and they expected me to be just calm and peaceful after a week to two weeks of noncommunication!

When I started praying more each day, I gave in and calmed

down. They can do their best taking care of Papa from their end, and I would just hope and pray for a miracle from my end. I became the committee on praying for miracles.

I had some money then, enough to last a few months, so I didn't bother looking for the next short job. I simply just went to the daily 8 a.m. Catholic mass about 2 long blocks away. I did my best to be there by 7:30 a.m. or even earlier because I had a couple of prayer books and all these numerous prayer cards with me and I was doing my best to recite them all!

It turned out that the daily Mass was only 30 minutes long. By being there early to pray before mass, I still spent a good hour inside the church. Once the mass was over, I recited a few more prayers, even as the priest and the volunteers had started turning the lights off. I got so much into reading my prayer cards that there were days when I looked up only to notice that everyone had left.

I think the most attendees for daily mass that I counted during those summer months was 45. It was not like a thousand churchgoers were there. Maybe I was the only one willing to pray all day long!

Then again, I admit that I was there because of a temporary need. I had a feeling that I was just going through a phase, that I will eventually slow down.

Before I went to church, I woke up at 6 a.m. I had an hour to prepare. My goal was to be out of my apartment by 7 a.m. I usually got out of my apartment by 7:15, and entered the church by 7:25. I was always disappointed, thinking I should be there earlier to pray more.

On Saturdays, I discovered that besides the 8 a.m. short, daily mass, the church had confession scheduled at 3:30 p.m., for 45 minutes, to 4:15 p.m., after which they had the 4:30 p.m. hour-long Sunday version of the mass. This mass is called an "anticipated" mass, which was mass celebrated on the eve before the actual day of obligation. I took these additional hours to be an opportunity for more time inside the church.

There were two churches near me. One was two blocks south, and the other one was three blocks north. On Sundays, I went to my daily church for the 8 a.m. mass, then I went north for the 10 a.m. mass. I discovered that about 5 people prayed the rosary right after the 10 a.m. mass, at 11. I joined them. I got out of church past 11:30 a.m.

I finally went to confession. I had not gone to confession for years, I didn't think it was necessary, and I had my own set of beliefs anyway. This time, I thought that confession would "cleanse my immortal soul," so that God would hear me better. I was desperate for Papa to have a miraculous cure.

The confessions at my church were face-to-face. They did not have a confessional that would had been a little more impersonal. I had become a familiar daily mass face anyway, there was no need for any concealment.

There were 3 priests who took turns saying mass and hearing confession on Saturdays. In time, all three of them had sat with me, had heard my confession and had known of my father's condition.

I deliberately memorized even more prayers. My rationale here was that it would be good to memorize as many prayers as I can because all this was new to me, I was very interested and willing, and all this might wane. There will come a time in a few months when I had to stop all this and start concentrating on my art and writing again. Because of Papa's condition, it was difficult for me to write or do art.

I will also once again have to find employment. All this religiosity was not permanent.

I felt that even if all this "fanaticism" waned, at least I should already have memorized the prayers, in case I wanted to say them in the future.

Early on, I discovered a word, "chaplet."

According to Wikipedia, "a Chaplet is a form of Roman Catholic prayer which uses prayer beads, but is not necessarily related to the Rosary. Some chaplets have a strong Marian element, others focus more directly on Jesus or the Saints. Chaplets are 'personal devotionals.' They have no set form and vary considerably. While the usual five-decade rosary is a chaplet, often chaplets have fewer beads than a traditional rosary and a different set of prayers."

I discovered that the rosary, where you recite the Hail Mary five times in groups of ten, which I had known how to do since grade school, is itself a chaplet. There were many chaplets!

In September, I discovered "The Divine Mercy Chaplet," which is recited using the rosary as a counting device. There was the basic Divine Mercy chaplet, but online there were additional verses. I was able to memorize everything by continuous repetition. Even when I walked on the streets, I was praying and repeating verses over and over.

"The Divine Mercy" refers to Jesus' blood and water that came forth when he was pierced by Longinus using a lance, to make sure he was dead before they took him down from the cross. The image of Jesus with a heart that has blue and red rays of light, representing water and blood, coming from His heart is the image of the Divine Mercy.

I also used my fingers to count the Hail Marys when I prayed the rosary while walking or taking public transportation.

At home, I prayed even more. I bought a booklet for praying the Stations of the Cross and prayed that at home. I also prayed the rosary at home.

I prayed in bed, staring at the ceiling, imagining that God was there, and I always fell asleep in the middle of some prayer. When I woke up, I tried to continue where I left off.

I memorized Psalm 23, The Magnificat, and The Divine Praises. You can Google these if you want.

Amel gave me a crucifix more than two decades ago. I never hung it anywhere. It was always on a table or shelf. I treated it like a teddy bear in bed. I clutched it, imagining connection with God and Papa. Papa was the one who gave me the simple, cheap rosary

I had been using. I clutched that as well in bed, because I prayed the rosary in bed. Usually I fell asleep doing it.

Catholics have this thing called a "scapular." The word originates from the scapula, or shoulders. In researching about this, I learned that there are two types, the large monastic scapular, which look like aprons worn by monks, nuns and other clergy and the small devotional scapular, which laypeople can wear. The devotional scapulars are those two squares of cloth, one placed on the chest and the other placed in the back, connected by cords hung on the shoulders.

Mama told me when I was small that those little squares were cumbersome to wear. There were two popular scapulars for laypeople. One is the brown and the other one is the green. I researched them. The wearer needed to be initiated into the brown scapular movement, while the green scapular can just be worn.

Here was another way to further my "fanaticism." Wearing any scapular needed willingness and dedication. Just wearing it for the heck would make it irritating and burdensome to do, but if I were really into it, I would be happy and willing to do it.

By November, I bought both brown and green scapulars. I approached the deacon of my church and asked him if there was anyone who can initiate me into the brown scapular movement. He said he would be honored and happy to do it. I showed him a prayerbook that had the initiation ceremony. Long story short, he put on his robe, read the prayer, blessed me with holy water from his bucket, called an "aspersorium," and sprinkled me with holy water using what looked like a mace, called an "aspergillum."

I was so thankful for what he did for me that when he asked me to show up in two weeks, to help feed the poor on November 28, Thanksgiving Day, I couldn't say no. Well, I was willing to do it. I thought it would be good for me.

Catholics are encouraged to make sacrifices to get closer to God. Some books and articles mentioned all these above as part of making sacrifices. I honestly never felt that doing any of these was difficult. None of these were sacrifices to me. I thought I was cheating because I was enjoying what I was doing.

On the other hand, I got into my interpretation of an imaginary zone of "needed practices" in order to get God to heal my dad. So I had this idea that I was "in the zone."

I felt I weakened this zone when twice I made plans to attend daily mass the next day and I overslept and missed them. I actually cried those days when I woke up. As I write this, I no longer feel this desperation, but way back then, it was just so important for me to do them for my dad that I felt so bad that I missed mass.

I want to tell you, my beloved reader, before I end this chapter, that all this above normal religiosity, including the time when I felt the vibrations in bed, and felt the scampering movements, was my period of 40 days and 40 nights.

CHAPTER 45

NEIGHBORS

My brother was nice enough to update me once in a while as to what had been going on, but each time he called me to give me negative updates, I felt that my praying, all that energy and time, was not enough. I needed to put in more effort. This is why I called my approach an experiment, calibration or tweaking.

I needed my brother's voice and updates, but I noticed that it was also weakening me, so it was good and bad. My illusion of miracles kept coming and going. Reality always took over. Like a balloon that wanted to float up into the sky, and just drift away with the clouds, my dream of being miraculous for my father was held down by twine, and each time anyone from Manila called me for updates, it felt like the balloon string was tied to someone's wrist.

☙

And then there was Dank, my neighbor downstairs. He was a black guy with nerdy glasses, a little overweight, and probably in his fifties. I did not think he worked. A lot of people in my neighborhood struggled. I thought he was one of them. He probably got a monthly check from the government, I figured, because on a regular day, he just sat on the steps or the porch of our apartment building. I never asked.

Like Papa, he had cancer. Unlike Papa, he was going through chemotherapy and nobody cared for him.

I noticed Dank got thinner in the face. He was still pear-shaped overweight.

I was affected and depressed because of Papa's condition, but here was someone nearby. I became sad and worried for Dank as well. I thought he was not eating, thinking that his health might affect his eating habits in a bad way.

I had eggs in my refrigerator, and I also made sure to have a regular supply. Each time I boiled two eggs for myself, maybe once a week, I boiled two more for Dank. I searched for him or asked Karen to open the first floor entrance to their hallway, and hung a shopping bag with the eggs in it on his apartment door knob.

Sometimes, he was at Karen's unit, so I joined them, gave him the hard boiled eggs and visited with them.

"Why do you keep giving me eggs?" he asked.

"Because I eat them myself, and I would not bring you cake, which would be more expensive. Eggs are cheap, easy to cook and safe to eat, and I am concerned about you not eating. My dad has cancer too," I explained.

He laughed and said thanks.

One time, I bought a few more prayer cards from the downtown church gift shop—the Sacred Heart of Jesus, St. Maximilian Kolbe, a patron saint of drug addicts, and St. Peregrine, who was the patron saint of cancer. I gave one of each to Karen and Dank.

෴

From 2010 to 2011, I studied hypnosis, neuro-linguistic programming, and hypnotic words, informally, yet intensively, at home. I watched video seminars, listened to audios and read books. I wanted to find out if and how my writing could improve with the use of hypnosis. I learned some techniques. I also learned about body language and gestures. Around that time, Terra was also my neighbor. She and Karen hung out a lot then.

One time, in 2011, Karen approached me, and said, "Terra told me you know hypnosis."

"I've been studying but only on my own; I'm not sure if I can hypnotize anyone," I said.

"Can you hypnotize me?" she asked.

"What for?" I asked.

"Oh, stuff," she said.

"I can look into that," I answered.

I remembered a couple of lessons that mentioned that an addictive personality remained addictive. The secret to curing addiction was to shift the addiction to something else. One hypnotist said that he made a cassette of his voice with messages of curbing the addiction, but he also gave the client a hypnotic suggestion to get addicted to the sound of his voice on the cassette. Then in time he weaned the client away from constantly listening to the cassette.

There was my weak point. I can't have a neighbor become addicted to my voice, however that would be done. I need more knowledge and research. I should attend seminars!

Then she said, "Well, I'm not ready to quit yet, but just in case I am, will you help me?"

I did not think she was ready to quit anything anyway. I had always thought that she was a nice neighbor though. I had visited with her and brought food to her.

I had seen Karen come up to me, still able to talk, but she swayed. She usually said she was drinking with friends somewhere downtown.

In more than one occasion, as she swayed, she groggily said, "Val, I wanna come up to your place to see how you're progressing with your porcelain dolls!" Leave it to Karen to make me feel like that girl with the glass menagerie.

But when she mentioned herself getting treated by a psychic surgeon and then telling me that Dank had cancer, I found a relevant connection with her and Dank.

ぴ

I was gone for two weeks, so I came home with my luggage, and Dank was outside, seated on the porch steps.

He looked okay, but he talked to me as if he knew that I knew he had cancer. Maybe Karen mentioned me to him. It was October 2013 and the weather was beginning to get cold.

He said he was just at the VA, doing his chemotherapy. He was supposed to be there for a few days, but he was taking a break and wanted to come home. He stuck out his tongue, saying it was red from the chemotherapy. He showed me his fingers and his fingernails. They were discolored, bluish, and much darker than usual.

I asked him if he was able to eat. He said he had to force himself to eat, he couldn't eat well, he had lost his appetite, had a hard time swallowing and he couldn't taste the food. He said weed made him just a little hungry. Without it, he did not care to eat at all.

I had been changing my attitude towards marijuana for a while then, because some documentaries indicated beneficial effects against cancer.

He showed me his shirt pocket, and it had a container that had a tube. He told me that the tube connected directly to his heart, and that was the chemotherapy. As he told me this, he also lifted his shirt, and out flopped his transparent plastic colostomy bag, and it wasn't empty.

He said he was going to hop on the bus soon to return to the hospital. It was still in the city, but it was all the way west of downtown Chicago. The nurses allowed him to leave for a few hours because he was one exceptional, robust, tough patient, he said. They were amazed that he was still strong and standing despite the chemotherapy he was doing.

I didn't remind him to pull his shirt back down. I was just glad I saw him. Colostomy bags should be opaque!

I thought it was providence for him to be the first person to greet me. He was not even supposed to be home. This prompted me to bring him eggs, take him to church once, and use my suspicious, experimental, hocus pocus psychic healing methods on him a few times.

I was experimenting, and my experiment not only involved the efficacy of the healing, but observing the reaction of the people

I encountered.

I exchanged phone numbers with him. I told him that I had been going to morning mass everyday, and if he wanted, he can walk with me and attend the 30-minute short weekday mass. He missed me a few times, and I said that was okay. We scheduled to go to Sunday mass together. He missed this too.

Finally, one day, we set an appointment for the morning mass the next day. The following morning I called him. He answered. We agreed to meet outside by the porch. It was still October.

I went out to the porch, and noticed it was drizzling a little. I had second thoughts about taking Dank because of the rain. I went back to my apartment to get my umbrella and a large black garbage bag that I can fashion for my head. He showed up. I gave him my umbrella and I held the black garbage bag on my head.

I walked slower than usual, but he still told me to slow down. I thought I was slowed down already. He had to catch his breath many times. It started to drizzle a little more.

We walked and talked with my head bowed down to fit the garbage bag. I saw his boaty old shoes get wet from the rain. He also seemed too weak to care about avoiding the puddles. His jacket pockets were jutting inside out. He didn't care to tuck them in. He clearly wasn't well. We reached the church.

As I saw him, I saw my dad. I wished it was Papa I was taking to church. In church, I sat next to him.

After mass, smiling, he stood up and looked up and around the church.

"This church is rich!" he said. He walked to a column. "Is this real marble? What can you steal from here?" he asked.

He told me he used to assist in Catholic mass when he was small. He told me he went to mass on a regular basis. What struck me was that if he did so, why was it the first time for him to set foot in this nearby church?

I felt bad for him. He was sick, but he was lucky to be going to the VA. I did not have medical insurance. I had to take care of my health, up until the time in the future when I will be financially stable enough from my art.

I knew the church was not rich. They had just announced their financial earnings a few times. I knew, because the previous week, I attended the Saturday 4:30 p.m. anticipated mass, and the Sunday 8 a.m. mass the following day.

I knew that the church needed money for a leaky roof. Some part of the dome above the altar was leaking down to where the bench was, where the priest saying mass sat down.

On our way home, we walked to the nearby grocery, Jewel, midway between home and the church. We walked in. I took a cart and pushed it for him. He mentioned that it's been a while since he was there, because he didn't want to get tired. That was how weak he was. Jewel was just a block away!

As we looked around at the produce section, it was early morning, we were talking, we had just gotten out of church, we were both distracted, that when we looked around, our cart was gone! We saw an old lady pushing our cart around, which had the umbrella and my balled up black garbage bag rain hoodie. We saw another unattended cart, which had a woman's medium sized black purse.

I approached the lady and, amused and smiling nicely at her, I asked if she was pushing the correct cart. She stared at the cart for a while and said sorry. She panicked a little, looked around for her cart and saw her unattended cart with her unattended purse. She rushed to it, apologizing, and making a comment that she almost lost her purse, money, I.D. and credit cards.

As Dank and I walked around again, he said, "If I'd been alone and not sick, I would already have left the store with that purse."

My God. Thank you. I stopped seeing my dad in Dank.

He finally bought some fresh fish and something else. I carried his grocery, and we slowly walked home.

☙

Early that year, before Papa got sick, I was waiting on the front porch for a package to be delivered by UPS. I ordered an electric guitar, an electric bass guitar, two amplifiers and some cords. They were the cheapest I can find. I wanted to play again, and I only had a classic guitar at home.

Out comes one of our building managers from the next building, where he lived. Our landlords owned adjacent buildings. I went next door to where he sat. I told him why I was outside, and he told me that some residents in my building had been losing their UPS and FedEx packages. They were delivered. Someone took them.

I was smiling and slightly amused, asking the building manager who he thought took the packages. With a nod and a mean stare, he pointed at Dank, who was just coming in through the gate from a walk.

I did my best to wait outside by the porch if I knew a package was arriving for me. UPS, FedEx and USPS have tracking systems online, it's easy to know when a package is already on their trucks and on its way to me.

The problem with everyone else was that they have regular jobs. They were bound to miss the trucks. The building managers are not obligated to receive packages for the residents.

When I wait for a delivery, I start waiting at 8 a.m. I sometimes waited from 8 a.m. to 4 p.m. for my packages to arrive. I did not live in a good area, and although we had the option to pick up packages at the FedEx and UPS warehouses miles away, I didn't drive. It was much smarter for me to just take out my folding chair, and sit on the porch with a book, a blanket if it's cold, a newspaper puzzle, a pen and a mug of coffee. Well, I didn't do this everyday anyway. There had been gang-related shootings on my block.

☙

One night, I was hanging out somewhere in Chicago, my phone rang. It was Dank. He asked me if I would want to check out a guitar his friend was selling. He said a brand. I said no thanks. I was at a bar, I didn't hear him well.

A few days later, I called him, to give him some hard-boiled eggs.

"Have you seen my place?" he asked. "Why don't you come down and see my place."

I said okay. I had the eggs, but I also decided to share with him my holy water. I asked if he had a container for holy water. When I got down, he opened his door. It smelled of weed. He should smoke because he had cancer. It was medical marijuana.

"I was wondering why you kept giving me eggs. I figured you haven't been to my place. Let me show you my food."

Our units were convertible studios, so even though we had small units, they were divided into two rooms. He led me to his second room, which was the kitchen area. He had shelves stacked with food! There were multiple boxes and cans of the same things, all perfectly stacked, with the labels all facing outwards. I wondered if he was obsessive-compulsive. Karen's place was messier than mine, but my place was a mess as well. I didn't care much about anything but my art supplies. His place was pristine! He had OCD!

If I got into smoking weed all day long, my place would be messier than even the state it was normally in!

He opened cupboards. More food, neatly arranged. He opened his refrigerator. More food. He pointed to the eggs. Eggs! Dozens of eggs!

"You didn't have to bring me those eggs!" he exclaimed.

"Well, yeah, but you lost weight, I thought you didn't have food," I answered. In my mind, I thought, if the apocalypse happened, and all the groceries were looted and emptied out, or if the zombie apocalypse happened, I knew I would knock on his door.

He pointed to every table, shelf and platform he had all over the place. He had candy everywhere, in crystal bowls and goblets.

"I even have candy all over the place so I wouldn't have to move if I get the munchies!"

I was amused.

"I actually wanted to give you some of my food, because I cooked some ribs and spaghetti and I was losing appetite, they're beginning to just have freezer burns. Here!" he said, as he opened the freezer door.

He took out some containers from the freezer.

"I cook, and I cook a lot at a time, and place them in containers so I can warm them up. I know how to cook. You probably don't cook at home! You want some spaghetti?" he asked.

"Okay," I answered.

"What about the ribs? You can have these."

"Okay."

"I also have some frozen breakfast sausages. Here you can have these," he said.

"Okay."

He took out some grocery bags and filled them up with some of his frozen food. He placed everything in the bags, and placed them on the kitchen table.

"Take them with you when you leave," he said.

He had three televisions in the first room, all of them were on, loud and on different channels.

"How many shows do you have to watch?" I joked.

"They're always on. I have to keep them all on," he said.

I showed him my bottle of holy water, and I said if he wanted, I can share some with him. I asked for an empty container. He gave me a small crystal goblet.

"Here, you can put it here," he said. I poured some holy water into the glass, but it occurred to me to just give him the bottle.

"You know, I'll just give you the bottle. I'm going downtown anyway, I'll just get another bottle and more holy water for myself," I explained. He thanked me.

"Where did you put that picture of Christ I gave you?"

"It's here somewhere." Dank took it from the side of a figurine.

"You know, you're supposed to display the picture where everyone, including your guests can see it as they walk in. There is supposed to be some type of blessing from God if you do that," I commented.

"Where do you think I should position it?" he asked. "Where do think it should go? How about here?" He pointed to a space on his corkboard.

He continued, "You know I felt better when you prayed over me that one time. I actually felt lighter. I want to tell you how grateful I am. You didn't have to bring me those eggs, but I appreciate the thought. I have relatives who come and are just wondering what they will get from me when I die from this cancer." I prayed over him once at Karen's.

"Well I don't want you to die. My dad has cancer. I don't want him to die. I'm not near him, he's in the Philippines. We're neighbors. I want you and my dad to live!" I said.

"Karen's been here, and she likes my couch and my leather chair and my pillows. This is how she is." Dank started to hug and squish his leather pillows one after the other. "This is how she just *loooves* my furniture and stuff. She's all *giddy* and *happy* while she's feeling for where I keep my money!"

I laughed.

"Open that door over there," he said, pointing to a door that probably led to storage space.

"Why?" I asked.

"Just open it," he said. I did. A bike.

"You want to have that bike? I just upgraded it. I put new paint on it, and new seats and everything, but now I'm sick, I can't bike," he explained.

"No. I think you should keep your bike. You'll need it for when you get better. You should look forward to getting better!" I said.

"Okay, So you don't want the guitar thing I called you about earlier? 'Coz I know you play the guitar," he said.

"I already have a guitar," I said.

"No, it's not a guitar," he said.

"I thought you said it was a guitar," I said.

"No. Here, look," he said. He reached for a small cube box and handed it to me.

It was a small cube box. It said eBow, Electronic Bow for Guitar.

"I don't want it. You can have it if you want," he said.

"I don't have the money to pay you for this. You wanted 40 bucks for it," I said.

"No, I'm giving it to you. If you can use it," he said.

"I think I can use it. I thought you said you were selling a guitar, not this," I said.

"Well, then, have it. You'll find some use for it."

"Okay thanks. Would you like me to pray over you right now before I go?" I asked.

He said yes. So I did. I asked him to sit on a chair.

I went behind him. I placed my hands on his shoulders. I prayed over him, two feet from his nearest loud television.

"Can you turn off the TVs?" I asked. I tried to concentrate. I wasn't vocalizing my visualization exercise, but the noise competed with my thoughts. Three loud TVs. Really. I thought that if he had OCD or something else, he might feel uneasy if he turned off his televisions. Turning three televisions on and off might be a hassle for him. He turned them all off.

I think I was silent for a good five minutes, maybe less, visualizing heaven opening up and sending him rays of healing light and energy, enveloping and passing through his body.

I was glad we had the time together.

I said goodbye and left him with my bottle of holy water and my prayers and good intentions. I looked at the picture of Jesus, properly displayed.

I was thankful. As I left with grocery bags filled with food he cooked, he lifted his shirt and once again his colostomy bag showed. I left with a few boxes of breakfast sausages and about 4 containers of frozen ribs and spaghetti he cooked. Two weeks later, I defrosted some of his food. They didn't taste right. I took food from someone whose tongue was red and had no working taste buds. I had to throw them out. Besides I really should also block out that image of the dangling colostomy bag out of my mind.

And the guitar contraption. It was brand new. That one cost $99 online. I looked it up the moment I got back to my apartment on the second floor. He was not able to figure out what it was, nor its use, nor the value of it. He didn't play the guitar.

I played the guitar, I had an electric guitar, an electric bass guitar, their amplifiers, and plugs. I just bought all these at one time, cheap, for a total of $350. They were the reason I waited on the porch for three days last May. The bass guitar got delayed and came on the third day.

I also had a classical guitar an uncle gave me about 20 years ago.

I never needed that small $99 dollar contraption he gave me. It's used for a later skill.

Before this collection of guitars, I had a better, earlier electric guitar which I gave to my brother.

Thanks Dank, my friend. I will keep the contraption. I cannot rat him out. I might give the thing to my brother who also had a few electric guitars, or I might put it on Ebay. God forgive me and my friend. I can't ask my neighbors who lost something like this thing in the mail.

As I end this chapter, I visualized Dank, in the near future, healthy and out on the porch. He sees each and every passing delivery truck, all with the sound of the musical bells of ice cream trucks. I really hoped he gets better soon.

CHAPTER 46

JACKS-OF-ALL-TRADE

This is the chapter I most dread writing. It is now February 22, 2014. Tomorrow, I turn 49. As I type this at 4:40 p.m. Chicago time, it is already my birthday in Manila.

It has been months. Whatever chapter I last wrote before I got my muse back was written in September 2013.

Papa was in and out of the hospital for what my brother and I considered incredible, seemingly stupid, spoiled reasons.

One night Papa prayed the rosary with Mama and Dinna. I'm sure Mama sat on a chair or on their bed, but Dinna probably knelt. They said Papa knelt and then sat in the common cross-legged position. The rosary consisted of 53 Hail Marys and a few other prayers.

By the time Papa tried to stand up, he was not able to. He lost sensation in one of his legs, and had to be hospitalized. His leg had to be rehabilitated for weeks! He should had just sat on a regular chair.

Then one time he went in for asthma. That also took more than a week. He also had a complaint that brought him to the family dentist a few times.

Each time he went in the hospital, Dinna and Mama stayed with him as well. Kuya Jing updated me once in a while, but Dinna and Mama weren't calling me at all. Oddly enough, Papa was not complaining too much about his cancer. He said it hurt a little sometimes.

Kuya Jing sold nutritional supplements, a multi-level marketing business with claims of improvements even on sick individuals. Some of his customers had testified that they became more active and healthier after taking the supplements.

Based on his experience with his supplements, he suggested for Papa to take a certain daily dose that might just combat cancer. It was not an exact science, but Papa was not too cooperative. Papa insisted on taking so much less.

Kuya Jing and I both finished a bachelors degree in Biology. We may not be doctors, but we both sensed that the amount Papa was taking was useless. I was all for what Kuya Jing was suggesting. Both of us figured that Papa had a chance if he followed a combination of our regimens scheduled to become complementary with each other.

My distance from all of them has put me in a place of idealism.

Meanwhile, they all seemed to counteract each others' methods. All of them had something to say about the others' characters. We seemed to be riding a lifeboat with a hole and everyone was telling everyone else who should stick his finger in the hole, even as the entire boat sank.

Dinna, Mama and I were the more religious people. Dinna was taking care of both Mama and Papa, so I felt the need to tackle Papa's disease through religion, becoming the most religious of all of us.

I had the luxury of going to church everyday and praying some more at home. I had no choice, because it was mental torture not to hear from them for weeks.

Whenever Dinna called, she claimed to always be tired from all the physical effort, appointments, chores and errands she had to do. I give her credit for her physical strain. It was not about me and my distress. I learned not to fault her for not calling me at all. She had the most immediate, most tiring input in this ordeal.

Amel stayed in Bohol with her family. She flew to Manila once in a while to check up on Papa, but she was busy herself. She had six kids and a spouse. All the kids went to school.

In October, Bohol had a massive earthquake. While Amel's

family and their home were lucky enough not to be badly hurt by the event—they were safe and their home wasn't damaged—the island lost lives, many homes and at least 11 historic, old churches. There were more than 100 sinkholes that resulted all over the island. Many roads shifted and became unusable.

Felix, Amel's husband, who was a book designer and artist, was affiliated with a prestigious family in Manila, who gave them a small amount of cash for supplies to buy and distribute to the local community. Over and above their family's well-being, Amel and Felix became busy helping the rest of their local community.

Kuya Jing updated me as often as he can, and for the most part, I listened to mentally draining updates and frustrations. While he was only two hours away from Manila, I worried about him driving to and fro. He was a great driver, had always been, but still.

Whenever Papa and Dinna called, they complained about Kuya Jing's unwillingness to spend time with them, to at least experience for a day the difficulty of caring for Papa and Mama.

Kuya Jing, on the other hand was in a bind himself. He had his own home, with bills to pay. He traveled to faraway locations promoting his business.

Papa really did not wish for me to be there, I was in Chicago. Kuya Jing was nearby. I was excused.

☙

When Lolo Jesus had a stroke, Dinna and I took care of him. Kuya Jing, Dinna and myself were still in college. Amel was still in grade school.

Kuya Jing had started living away from us. Even though he did not have to, he took some semesters in another location, about 80 kilometers, or 50 miles away, so he stayed in a dormitory most of the time. You really cannot judge travel time in Manila by the miles because of congestion.

Dinna and I kept Lolo Jesus company. We slept in his room, which became Papa and Mama's room years later, when they remodeled it.

When Lolo needed a bath or needed to use the bathroom, it was I who took him there. I bathed him in the tub and I wiped and washed him with soap and water after he pooped. I held my breath as he used the toilet. It was a sacrifice I did without complaints.

My concern and love for my grandpa spanned years, more beyond those months of his recovery from a stroke. When he felt rejected by his kids at one point in time, when I was still in high school, I opted to be with him on Lubang Island as soon as school was out. I bought and brought all the books I can read and stayed with him on the island away from Manila's comforts, television and electricity. I saw him sit on a folding chair every afternoon, staring at the darkening sky, quiet, drinking his bottle of beer for the night.

☙

Papa mentioned my efforts once in a while, because now it was Dinna who was stuck doing it for him. While he complained about Kuya Jing not having done it even once, he mentioned what I did in the late '70s to early '80s for Lolo Jesus, a way to tell me that he appreciated what I did in the past.

In my mind, I was not any better than my brother. I left. I had no plans to return. I wrote memoirs to prove that I'm still a good person, despite the absence of the people I should be around with.

I looked for razor-sharp, stinging slivers of salvation in short bursts of interaction. I'm sorry, that sentence just came to my mind.

I wrote to preserve my own sanity and humanity.

The doctors only prescribed pain medication for Papa. Papa, Mama, Dinna, Kuya Jing and Amel all agreed to only have him take the pain medication when Papa was in pain.

The good news was that Papa never really fully felt pain. The doctor prescribed for him to take the pain pills once every 6 hours, but they told me that they successfully managed to only give it to him once every 8 to 10, or even 12 hours. Papa and everyone else with him claimed that he never was in serious pain. The doctors he saw all wondered why he was not suffering.

Maybe that was the best miracle God can grant us for the meantime.

One of the doctors who diagnosed him with pancreatic cancer had a wife who recently died of pancreatic cancer. She suffered. When the doctor sat Papa and Dinna down to tell them that he was sure it was pancreatic cancer after tests and scans, he was sad and close to tears, having just gone through the suffering and death of his wife. He and some other doctors had become friends of my family through the years. For the next few months, he wondered why Papa was not in pain.

The dentist also had a relative who died of pancreatic cancer. He too wondered why Papa was not suffering.

☙

One day in mid November, Kuya Jing called me. He said Papa was going back to the hospital for "pain management." What this meant was that Papa's pain was finally kicking in, and they might have to start dripping morphine into his system. What this also meant was that Papa might never get to come back home again. He will eventually die.

What this meant to me was that I needed to even double my praying efforts. I was now even more desperate that some form of great miracle should happen. I still believed that he will just one day hop off the hospital bed healthy, despite his morphine drip.

I once saw an interview of a prominent Catholic priest, who had also written books, on YouTube. On the purpose of healing miracles, he said that it was not for the purpose of physical healing that God allowed it once in a while. It was for the purpose of strengthening faith and the salvation of the soul that such things happen.

I felt that the faith of each individual member of our immediate family might be faulty, but still stronger than average. The healing miracle that I was asking for was just icing on the cake. None of us would get mad at God for allowing our beloved father to die.

※

Kuya Jing called me again. He had been calling me almost on a daily basis. He was with Papa. They were next to the speakerphone, so they both were able to hear me. Mama and Dinna were away, to run some errands and do some grocery shopping. Kuya Jing had to be with Papa at home. They were also waiting for Amel to arrive from the airport.

I asked Kuya Jing to sit Papa on a chair, and I'll do some healing on him. I told Kuya Jing to imagine Jesus Christ, to say out loud, "Lord Jesus Christ, please appear to me in human form," and when he started to imagine Jesus Christ as being in the room with them, to let me know.

He said, "Okay."

I said, "Next I will guide you to touch Papa where I feel he should be touched."

I asked Papa, "Papa, are you in pain right now?" He said yes.

I said, "Okay, remember this pain and Kuya Jing and I will make you feel better."

I told Kuya Jing to touch Papa on his head with his two hands. Touch him on his shoulder. Touch him on his left and right brow. Touch him on his knee. Go in front of Papa and kneel and touch his feet with his palm. Then touch him just behind the knee.

Then Amel arrived, and once again I explained this to Amel and asked her to do the same thing and replace Kuya Jing. What was funny about Amel was that she wanted to stop. Later on she did, refusing to follow me.

She had become a born again Christian years back. She had been telling Mama and Dinna to stop praying to the Virgin Mary, that it was wrong. I too would be wrong. I had a feeling she would want to stop. I thought it was funny. I wanted to see how far she would do whatever I told her before she became uncooperative.

What was funny about Amel, she edited my first book. She edited the Lessons from a Psychic Surgeon chapters. She knew what I was up to, but her Christian interpretations had changed.

I felt the connection with God, when Papa and Kuya Jing were alone. As I was asking my brother to touch Papa, it was, in a way, the moment I got Kuya Jing to honor and serve Papa. This was the precious time they had together.

Papa claimed that his pain had dissipated. I told him this was what I had been trying to teach them all along. They just did not want to listen to me.

Dinna months ago agreed to learn this, but I never heard opposition nor a glimmer of interest in it. All she said was that she did it. Her answers, whenever I asked, had the flavor of blah.

I spent three decades of an uncomfortable shift in my belief system because of the healing lessons I got from the psychic surgeon. I opted to leave and not take them to where I was going, to forget all this because its impact was great, but back then it was pulling me the opposite way. I opted not to tell them anything, because I did not want their own realities to blur, and because they might look for the psychic surgeon in Manila. I thought that what I had chosen to leave, they might find attractive.

I doubted Dinna made any difference.

As I prayed for miracles for Papa over so many months, sometimes I asked the angels to pay him a visit. I joked with God and prayed to make all the members of my family, from myself to my parents, to my siblings and to my nieces and nephews to all become miraculous themselves—I thought it would be funny for them to discern and display strange things themselves.

Dinna, with her statements to me of late, seemed to have noticed strange things that she was unwilling to share with me.

☙

There was a passage in the Bible when Jesus said all the world will listen to his message, except where he was born. I'm just paraphrasing. I had always remembered this. The psychic surgeon said the same thing at one point. It was easier to convince strangers than to convince family.

To visualize the healing of a family member while remembering past conflicts is a great challenge. To say, "Leave it to God to decide for us" is so much easier. Add the uncertainty of whether or not the healing did work.

Then what if Papa did heal, life would return to normal. Maybe there is also fear in returning to normal. Maybe it was time for a change. Maybe Papa did have to go.

All this just seemed like an impossible feat. We're all kidding ourselves one way or another.

It was during this time of my heightened religiosity that I made the pain go away not just for Papa, but for that worker with the pins in his knee and elbow as well. I knew I can do something, but maybe it was not yet enough.

∽

Back to that day. Everyone but myself converged to take Papa to the hospital. Imagine this again—Papa was leaving home for good. There was even more desperation and sadness in the air.

I asked a simple but ridiculously sounding request over the phone—for Amel to touch Papa as I wanted to touch him had I been there. She refused. The refusal was easy. She looked to God her own way. She did not even try to humor me for a few minutes. Not that I blamed her. I was not really in my right mind, or was I? Who would believe in faith healing, psychic healing or psychic surgery? My desperation was my own.

∽

In hindsight, Papa also held a grudge with us. As far as I was concerned, I left him to become my own free self. He never permanently left that house. When I was in college, he wanted me and my brother to pursue medicine. We both "changed our minds." We cannot be stopped. In his mind, the word to use was "refuse." Refuse we did. Why would he listen to us before he listened to his doctors? They had given him the go signal to die. It was good enough for him.

While I was feeling uncertain about my future, and I thought pursuing art was only a pipe dream, when I was still in college, I had a class in ecology. My professor was highly into seaweed farming. I described to him the location of a secluded beachfront property we had on Lubang Island, how it was situated in relation to the open sea, and how the waves behaved. The professor got excited about the place. He said it might be conducive to seaweed farming. I told Papa I was willing to return to the island to see if I can farm seaweed. He refused and never wanted to hear it. I kept at it for more than a year. I decided to leave the Philippines. Anywhere but there. Here was one factor that made me leave.

When he got sick, Kuya Jing and I researched about alternative forms of treating cancer, especially since the doctors told him that his case, due to his age and health, was no longer treatable and that the best they can give him were pain pills. Papa, despite the fact that he knew he was dying, gave subtle hints that he didn't really want to hear about our so-called treatments.

My brother sold nutraceuticals. They were effective. I researched about the ingredients myself. My brother and I talked about tweaking the dosage as we observe his progress. There was no progress. Papa only took half at the most of what Kuya Jing said was to be the effective dose.

Papa seemed to want to die, if only to punish his kids, I thought. Or maybe he was ready. Life was over. He was 80 years old.

☙

If there was anything I owed Papa, I inherited his being the Jack-of-All-Trades, Master of None. I love my existence, albeit more challenging in many ways—mentally, emotionally, geographically, financially, spiritually.

For myself, I made sure that as I became a jack-of-all-trades, I mastered each of my trades more and more. I never abandoned an interest to move on to the next one. I made sure I only placed my varied interests in my mental back burner. I kept all my kindling lit, each one of them ready to start a creative fire.

This is why I am a writer. This is why I am an artist. This is why I composed *Dollman the Musical, A Memoir of an Artist as a Dollmaker,* filled with songs and verses. And now, this is why I claim to be a healer, still with reluctance, still not good yet, but here I am.

This was how I had been honoring him all through these decades, despite the fact that once in a while he and I argued over the phone.

He composed one song and produced it. He got a band and a singer to sing it. He had piano pieces printed. His song was entitled *Unfaithful Sweetheart.*

When I was in first grade, he paid my music teacher to spend time with me to teach me piano in the school's music room. I stared at the piano's black and white keys, not really knowing what I was doing. The teacher was intent on teaching me the mechanics, but she and Papa should have introduced the heart of the activity first.

The same thing happened when Papa brought Kuya Jing and I to our distant cousin to teach me bass guitar, while Kuya Jing learned lead guitar. Nowadays, I wished Papa showed us a live band, and explained to us why bass guitar was just as important as lead guitar. I thought he just wanted me to play second fiddle to my older brother, as usual.

When he enrolled my brother and I to Saturday morning martial arts classes in school, where there were only 8 to 12 of us students from a school of 2,000 students, we were all barefoot as we learned what 2,000 students from the school passed up, I was just conscious about my wide-sized flat feet. I thought the rest of the student population was enjoying their lives, comfortably watching Saturday morning cartoons at home. I missed the heart of the martial arts class. I never thought it was an honor and a privilege to study those barefooted moves.

I did not see the reason why he took Dinna, Kuya Jing and I to the Yamaha Music School to learn to play the keyboard, when he could not afford to buy an organ for the home. There was an upright piano owned by his mother, but grandma only bothered to have it tuned once, when we were still small. We were forbidden to touch it.

I only found the heart in college when Papa enrolled Dinna and I to speedreading school. Kuya Jing and Amel followed suit later. Only when I appreciated speedreading school, did I find the heart in the rest of everything else we did to learn great, wonderful things—trades—beyond school.

❧

The deacon who enrolled me in the brown scapular movement about two weeks before Thanksgiving requested for me to show up for the annual Thanksgiving Day feeding of the poor. They needed help serving turkey and all the trimmings to the poor in the community at noontime, right after the 11 a.m. mass. It was to be held in the school lunchroom.

It was my first time to help feed the poor. I was very happy with the neat ceremony the deacon did for me, that I cannot refuse him. I thought it would be good for me because it will be a new experience and since I was writing this book anyway, I might be able to also have a story from that experience.

This request from the deacon was about two weeks prior to the event, Thanksgiving Day, which was on November 28, 2013. I remember going to two more confessions on two consecutive Saturdays prior to the week of Thanksgiving. I told both priests that I was looking forward to being a server at the Thanksgiving luncheon.

❧

It was about a week before Thanksgiving when Kuya Jing, and then Dinna and Papa called me to tell me that Papa was going to the hospital for pain management. I suddenly got the thought that he might not come back home. He was going to get worse.

&

On the Wednesday before the Thursday that was Thanksgiving Day, which was November 28, 2013, I was told that Papa was dying. He was no longer capable of movement and speech but he can still hear and understand. However, it might still be a few days before he passed away.

Earlier that week, Robert, who bought my first ever group of porcelain dolls, called me and asked if I wanted to hang out on Wednesday night, the eve of Thanksgiving. I told him I did. I thought I needed a break. Robert knew that I had been going to church for Papa. That night he picked me up and we went to a bar to see a friend of his sing with a band. I had pizza and a drink.

Robert took me home. I took a few pictures of the band on my cellphone and emailed the pictures to my brother. I had gotten back into music, and in a way I was trying to get my brother to get to playing his guitar again.

I had been practicing this cheesy Filipino song from the '80s, *Hindi Ako Iiyak,* on my electric guitar and on my classical guitar, because I had always loved it, playing the two professionally recorded versions of the song on YouTube every once in a while. The song's title means "I Won't Cry." It's really about someone who is missing his spouse, since they had just separated. The chorus had more general verses. "Don't you worry, I won't cry. I won't feel bad, I won't shed a single drop of tear. The love that I once felt from you, for someone like me, so undesirable, is enough."

Now I was learning it on the classical guitar as my second serious song. A month before that, I had already memorized my most favorite song, *Moon River* by Henry Mancini. I had hoped to play both songs for Papa, to hint that if he died, I will not be sad.

I was never able to show him that I had lately begun to play the guitar again. I did not tell anyone that I bought cheap guitars and amplifiers. I had planned to resell them in case I got cash strapped anyway.

When Robert brought me home on Wednesday, Thanksgiving Eve, after pizza, a beer and seeing his friend sing and perform with his band, it was about 10:00 p.m., Chicago time.

As soon as I walked in, my brother called from the hospital to tell me that Papa was dying, but was still able to hear and understand. He said I can talk to him through the phone, and he will put it up close to his ear so that I can tell him whatever I wanted to tell him in confidence, and no one else will overhear it.

"Okay, you can talk to Papa now," said my brother.

I rattled it all off. That I loved him and that I was in America not just to pursue my own ambition, but that this is what God wanted me to do. I told him I wanted to bring prestige back to all of our ancestors before us. I told him that soon I will become a famous artist and writer, and our last name will become known.

I told him that I had been praying for him to get well, and miraculously get cured, that I believed in miracles and I had strong faith in God, and that I know for sure that I was in God's good graces, but in case God decided to get him, that's okay as well.

I told him that despite all our arguments I love him so much, and that I would be honored to have him again as my father in case God decided to reunite us again on earth.

I told him that when he comes to see all of our ancestors and loved ones and friends, to tell them that I'm still here struggling to keep my ambition, because I had promised them all that one day I will trace all our relatives and friends and take care of them, as soon as my art starts to make money.

I told him I was here doing my best, pursuing my ambition, and that my success will come soon. Tell everyone he sees that I love them all, especially all my aunts and uncles and grandparents. I told him not to worry about us when he gets to heaven. I told him I will always love him.

Kuya Jing talked again and asked me if I was done. He said they will call again later. It might still be hours or a day more before he passed away. His phone needed to be charged.

I said okay. I put my cellphone down and charged mine as well.

I sat down and played my classical guitar. I played *Hindi Ako Iiyak*. I was practicing.

☙

My brother called and I instinctively looked at my computer's clock. It was a fateful 1:11 a.m. It was Thanksgiving Day. I saw repeating numbers.

"Hi Kuya Jing!"

"Val, we just want to let you know that Papa died about 30 minutes ago. We just were not able to call you then. I hope you understand."

"That's okay, Kuya, I'm okay. Can I talk to Mama?"

"Okay, here she is."

"Val!"

"Hi Ma, are you okay?" I asked.

"I was holding his hand, and he held mine, and then later on, he seemed to have stopped grabbing on to me. So I asked, Pablo, how come he's no longer holding me back? I guess that's when he passed," she explained.

"Mama, I just want to tell you that I have never prayed so hard for anyone, as much as I had spent for Papa. I want to tell you right now, I had come to realize that Dinna and I don't have kids. No one will ever pray to God this hard for us as much as I have for Papa. Just in case you go next, you make sure to come pick up Dinna and I when it becomes our turn to die. But for now, you should be okay. I need you to recover and be healthy. I'm not successful yet. I can't have you to go yet," I said, sad. My eyes teared up, my voice started to get hoarse, but I controlled myself. I didn't want to cry.

"Don't worry, Val. I won't. I love you," she said, She was sad.

"I love you too," I said back.

I talked to the other people in the room as well. Papa's last sibling standing, Tito Pablo, was someone I had not talked to in a long time. We exchanged a few sentences. I said there we were again. When Tito Nick died in the late '80s, I will mention his violent death in another book, Tito Pablo and I were on the phone crying. No thanks to late '80s technology, my phone bill that month was $1,000 plus. This time we didn't cry, but it seemed like deja vu all over again.

I also talked to some of my nieces and nephews.

ಲ

When I put the phone down, I talked, as if Papa can hear me, as if he was visiting. I told him I had been practicing a song I wanted to play for him, to show him that I had again found interest in playing the guitar. As I talked, I picked up my classical guitar, the one Mama's brother, Tito Nimitz, gave me more than two decades ago.

I played two songs I had wanted him to hear. *Moon River* and *Hindi Ako Iiyak*. I sang the songs, adding "Papa," where I found appropriate, thinking I was lightly humoring him, just in case he was really there with me. I was showing him I was okay, that I was happy in a way. I'm sure he is with God and everyone else I had been asking to intercede—the Virgin Mary, the saints, the angels.

ಲ

The next morning, Thanksgiving Day, I made sure to go to the 9 a.m. mass. They announced days before that there will be no 8 a.m. mass. There will be the 9 a.m., followed by another one at 11 a.m., followed by the feeding of the poor.

I went to the 9 a.m. mass, then went home, took a shower and went back for the 11 a.m. mass. Then I and most churchgoers went to the next building.

I was given a clean, white apron and a nametag.

I put the clean, white apron on. I was ready to serve the poor.

The lady found it difficult to spell my name, so I took the permanent marker and wrote on the nametag: VAL ZUBIRI.

Someday, everyone will be able to spell it correctly. All for you and our ancestors, Papa, and the rest of the world.

Ironic that Papa died on my Thanksgiving Day, I was celebrating it, but the rest of the family was in the Philippines, taking care of Papa's cremation. The Philippines does not celebrate Thanksgiving.

I socialized and served food to the poor. Some of them were just churchgoers from the 11 a.m. mass, but some were definitely poor, and some smelled of alcohol.

Then by 3 p.m. I went home with some leftover food. Papa always asked me if I was eating or if I had food to eat. I made sure I did.

Happy Thanksgiving, Papa. Happy Thanksgiving to all my loved ones whom I kept missing as I stage this illusion of my own humanity.

Goodbye Papa. We all loved you. We still do. This is how I honor you. In a book that will stay on forever on the shelves of others, and in my heart living a life as a Jack-of-All-Trades and Master of Everything, just like you. With all my prayers, dreams and good intentions that continue to grow.

*

In December, Dinna called me to assure me that even as all of them were in the room, no one else heard what I told Papa. Tito Pablo, Papa's brother, was there too. Amel and her kids had flown in the day before. They got a second room in the hospital for all of them to sleep in. That day in December, Dinna and I caught up with our stories. She was feeling better. She told me that as I talked, Papa's closed eyes produced a tear. When Papa died, Amel's kids sang religious songs of praise.

*

Once in a while, I would play my guitar and sing to my dad. I put in "Papa" wherever I can put it, and smile.

*

Don't you worry, Papa,
I won't cry, Papa
I won't feel bad, Papa
I won't shed a single drop of tear, Papa
The love that I once felt from you, Papa
For someone like me, so undesirable and unworthy, Papa
is enough.

☙

We're after the same rainbow's end, Papa
Waiting 'round the bend, Papa
Moon River, and me, and you, Papa.

Chapter 47

Providence

I was at a church when this Gospel was read.

A blind man approached Jesus and asked to see again. Jesus did the following: Using his "spittle," or spit, he wiped it on the man's eyes. Jesus then asked the man if he can see. The man said that he saw people but they looked like trees moving about. So Jesus did the same thing again, putting his spit on the man's eyes. He asked again. This time, the man said he was able to see clearly.

That was great coincidence. Providence again? I told of an earlier story, about the faith healer who healed Papa when he was young. Papa was dying of a lung infection due to a broken rib he got from falling off of a horse. After touching him, and pus poured out of him, the lady faith healer looked at *Lola* Tesay ("Grandma Tesay"), or Papa's *Tia* Tesay, ("Aunt Tesay") and pretty much did the same thing that Jesus did to the blind man.

After treating Papa, the healer turned to Lola Tesay, who wore thick eyeglasses, and the healer asked Lola Tesay if she wanted to get rid of her glasses, and see clearly.

Lola Tesay said yes. The same treatment was done to her. Lola Tesay said the healer spit directly on her eyes.

The healer asked the same question, if she can see better. Lola Tesay said yes, but it was still blurry. The healer once again did the same thing, From that time onwards, when Lola Tesay died when she was ninety, she had 20/20 vision except when she needed reading glasses.

The way it happened to Lola Tesay, as she described it to me years later, in the '80s, and with hesitation and the look of fear and astonishment, it was like when a person had dust or an eyelash in his eye and needed someone to blow quickly into the eye, to dislodge it. Except that the lady spit lightly into each of her eyes.

I asked who the lady was and how they got in touch with a healer. She did not want to elaborate.

I had always seen Lola Tesay as someone older, even when I was small. She was Papa's father's sister, who married late. She said she only married and became Lolo Milio's second wife, just for companionship. She had always been very superstitious and never liked the dark. She never talked about why she was always super-scared about stuff.

I tried to ask her more questions. Papa's parents had died. She claimed to be the only one left to have known the lady, and it's all in the past. Whoever that old lady was, she said, had already passed on. Maybe that was it. Respect and fear of the encounter. I would not call it "unknown." We acknowledge these things to happen, not regularly, but they happen. Healing happened during the time of Christ, and it happened to her and Papa.

In hindsight, suddenly getting 20/20 vision from the healer may had been one of Lola Tesay's more shocking events in her early life. Maybe she too went through a soul-searching odyssey. Maybe that inspired her to finish her degree, even though she was way past the age of an average college student.

※

I was out of town, spending time with some people for some reason that I would later describe in another book. We got to talking about belief in God and the paranormal.

I described to the guy, a religious and smart black guy who was younger than I was, events that happened, when I was with the psychic surgeon, and how the lady went into a trance.

I learned a lesson from him. A way to be able to shut up about supernatural occurrences.

He said, that these supernatural things do happen, but I should view my relationship with God as if God were my spouse. God does things to all of us that are sometimes best left unsaid.

This is how spouses should behave, lest they incriminate their own spouses and maybe even themselves.

Learn to keep things secret if they are supposed to be secrets. That way, no one gets in trouble.

I owe and thank him for that comment, one of the most memorable tips I had heard in a good while.

You, the reader, should as well.

☙

I'm going to tell you something that you will find out anyway. When I was still in the practice of checking out the Paranormal / UFO section of Borders Bookstore, when Borders was still open in downtown Chicago, my sister Amelia told me that there was this new thing called the "Bible Code." She explained it a little, but she wanted me to get the book and find out what it really was.

I saw the book, *The Bible Code* by Michael Drosnin. I didn't buy it then. I wasn't curious enough. I didn't really care for it then, I did not know what it was all about.

When 9/11 in 2001 happened, the Bible Code and Nostradamus' prophecies gained attention again. I finally understood what my sister was talking about when some documentaries on television featured it. Skeptics said that the believers of the Bible Code and Nostradamus always naturally found what they wanted to see, but it's all random.

I thought it would be nice to find my name using the Bible Code. Even then, there really was nothing I can do about the Bible Code because whatever computer program they possessed, it stayed with the researchers.

According to Wikipedia, "The Bible code, also known as the Torah code, is a purported set of secret messages encoded within the Hebrew text of the Torah. This hidden code has been described as a method by which specific letters from the text can be selected to reveal an otherwise obscured message. Although Bible codes have been postulated and studied for centuries, the subject has been popularized in modern times by Michael Drosnin's book, *The*

Bible Code, and the movie, *The Omega Code*."

What happened was that this "postulation for centuries" finally became possible with the invention of computers. The researchers were able to search for messages at computer speed.

The most popular method to see codes in the Bible is ELS, "equidistant letter sequencing," where meaningful words are discovered when letters get picked by the computer program as it skips a certain number of other letters. I'm sure they are researching other formulas to obtain letters.

Skeptics have also said that even the novel, *Moby Dick* can produce seemingly prophetic messages, so the Bible Code might just be a flight of fancy, an overly speculative program. You will find the words that you want to find. What you want to see is what you will get.

In 2012, about 10 years later, I looked for the Bible Code online. Finally, a website shared a version of the Bible code program online, using grids of the English Bible. I believe they are using the St. James version. DivineCoders.com had an online Equidistant Letter Sequencing program for everyone to check out.

I checked out "Val" and "Zubiri" and a few other words related to me. Only the Book of Chronicles contains both "Val" and "Zubiri." Actually, the nicknames of my other relatives were there too. There is supposed to be a Chronicles 1 and a Chronicles 2 in the Bible. I think DivineCoders.com put both books together.

Understandably, I thought "Valentino" was too long to be there. I had the longest name in school. I had the most syllables of any name in school in Manila.

Good, honest words were there to, like "fame," "book," "art," and "write," but so were the bad ones. "Hoax" is present. For skeptics, these words can also be found in the other books of the Bible.

I did not bother to find out other words relative to where my name was. I would say, I'm a skeptic myself, but it was novel to find my last name, and to find it only in the Book of Chronicles.

Oops, upon reading Wikipedia, just now, to mention the

definitions in this book, it occurred to me that I should also have looked for the reverse, "I-R-I-B-U-Z." I don't want to bother. I emailed the website, DivineCoders.com to Amel when I discovered it in 2012. She never emailed me any discoveries she may have made. She and her family, between the time when I hung out at Borders and 2012, had switched from Catholicism to Christian, but I don't know what denomination they are.

Those scholars have time to spend searching for meaning using the Bible Code, or Torah Code. I saw my name, I thought it was neat. I still have to continue pursuing my art and writing. If I do something substantial for the world in the future, maybe the scholars and hobbyists will bother looking for more messages related to me.

Because of the theme of this book, I had to add this in. At the very least, it will probably add to my mystique in the future.

Then again, I also saw my other family members there as well. I think the website used the St. James English version of the Bible. I could be wrong. What about the Catholic version? What about other languages? What about the Torah? And how is our name spelled in Hebrew or any other language? Obviously, there are many possibilities here. Remember too that there have been ancient books that were not included in the Bible, and I think the Torah.

For now, maybe you would want to go to the website before they decide to remove the program in the future. They had a downloadable version for your computer. See if your computer is compatible.

Look for you name. If your name is too long, like mine, look for your nickname. It would be neat to find your name or names there.

CHAPTER 48

CARING

In the news, there had been investment bankers and related individuals who had been somehow "accidentally dying" or "committing suicide." Conspiracy theorists online have been talking about this as if those financial professionals were murdered. The highest questionable claim I found online was a total of 20 people from all over the world.

I care about the world's economy, I wanted to shift my course to business or economics decades ago. I just was not able to. After Biology, I studied Mathematics. Then I did art. I have yet to connect art to business and economics. I think there's a way.

I have been praying for the economy to get better since 2008 when it tanked. In 2011, I learned that bankers and investors also committed suicide around 2008, even earlier than 2013 and 2014. While I only have a little money on my person, these people had prestigious jobs when they were alive. They had cars and expensive food and wine that I can only look forward to in the future. Yet I never envied them, I just wished all of us found ways to better ourselves.

What I noticed was wrong with me was that while I did not have the guts and stomach to ask people for money so that I can pay the rent and continue with my art, I looked forward to a successful future when I would be able to give away money to the causes that I felt strongly about. My grandparents kept telling us that our family was the envied one. They said we were "Royal Blood," as a joke. Hmm. My ancestors did come from Northern Spain.

Whatever the case, it was ingrained in our minds early on, that we were already somewhere on top. Envying other people was never a thought.

※

I lived in a bad part of the north side of Chicago. In 2008, the economy took a really bad fall. I lived on the block that had a nice-looking Baptist church that had a homeless shelter program in place. Just about every afternoon, there were lines to get in and spend the night on their lower floor. I wished I had a million dollars to give to that church.

I was working on my balcony one afternoon, sanding my bisque stage porcelain doll parts, when I suddenly heard the sound of what I thought were tractors, with echoes bouncing around the buildings. My balcony faced the alley, not the street. I wondered why the sound of tractors only lasted a few seconds. If there was work to be done, the ruckus should continue. It turned out that the sound came from gunshots. Four people standing on the sidewalk where the Baptist church was were gunned down.

The two nearby Catholic churches I had been going to needed money because one had leaks, and both of them had already gone over their budget for snow removal this last winter season. Winter was brutal. They also have charitable projects in place.

One of the two churches just successfully raised money for a cheaper crown for their Virgin Mary statue, after someone stole the previous, more expensive one.

The house next door to my apartment is actually a nonprofit. They have breakfast coffee and food on weekday mornings. One poor alcoholic person was found dead one morning at the front of the house.

※

In the Philippines, there were two calamities last year, in October. A supertyphoon, known to the world as Haiyyan, and known as Yolanda in the Philippines, was the worst typhoon to hit the country. Thousands were killed and thousands more were rendered homeless.

My mother comes from the island of Bohol. Bohol had the

worst earthquake ever, and at least 11 churches were totally demolished. These churches need to rebuild literally from the ground up. The adjacent island of Cebu also had some damaged churches.

200+ people died from the earthquake. The entire island population was affected. I wished I can help them. I have relatives whose houses collapsed. One of Mama's brothers was trapped in his house and firefighters and volunteers had to extricate him. Luckily he was not hurt. The house now will be demolished and the rubble will be donated to the church across the street, to be used as landfill. My other uncle, who owns the property, the one who gave me his classical guitar almost 3 decades ago, will have a smaller house built.

The best I can do was pray, but although Jesus said He can rebuild churches in a few days, I know Filipinos and the rest of the world aren't waiting for that to happen. They would do their best to rebuild the churches the physical way, with money and cement. I thought it would be nice to help in the efforts by selling my art in the 7 and 8 figures. Duh. My goal really hasn't changed. This has always been my goal. It's a matter of time. It might take decades. Maybe tomorrow.

Well, actually, when Jesus Christ said he will rebuild his temple in three days, he was referring to Himself resurrecting on the third day. I just recently got reminded of this explanation in a Catholic video. I heard this decades ago.

֍

Michael's Arts and Crafts Store on Belmont and Clark was the nearest art and craft supply store for me; I went there to buy most of my art supplies. They always had a "40% off for one item" coupon online, which I always printed out, and from spring to fall, for some years, I normally rode my folding bike to the store as often as I needed so many items. I did my best to use the 40% off coupon by buying only one item per visit.

One thing I liked about Michael's, they close at 9 p.m. It is located in Boystown, which is one of two gay areas in Chicago. The other gay area is called Andersonville, which people call

"Mandersonville." Figure that one out. I lived in Uptown, about 20 blocks north. I enjoyed biking to Michael's.

Every night at around 7 p.m., there was an outreach van that parked on the side of the Michael's building. Homeless teens congregated there, some of them looking too young to be in any bars in Chicago. Most of them, young men and women, were obviously gay. They looked nice, they smiled, they were with one another. They were homeless.

I researched online about homeless youth and young adults, and I discovered that a disproportionately huge number of them happened to be gay, lesbian, transgendered, bisexual, or whatever you might want to add in the mix.

Here is a trend. According to articles and videos online, as an increasing number of celebrities come out and get praised in the media for their courageous move, an increasing number of younger and younger ordinary people have also been coming out to their families, schools, communities and even churches.

More and more have been getting rejected and thrown out of their homes. Others run away. They come to Chicago, thinking they will find shelter and solace here.

With the harsh cold weather, which Chicago had been getting lately, this is the hell. This is where these young people with great potential get thrown out to—literally where there is gnashing of teeth. The people and the outreach truck have kept me inspired to push my art and writing further.

There is no "One day, I will help them." They need help now. Their families, peers, churches, schools and communities need to realize that only God, the Master, can condemn us human beings. We are not God.

I threw out my own sister Dinna once, just because we had a fight. I threw out someone else another time for another reason. I will gladly burn in hell. I deserve it.

☙

In 1996, I got featured on Chicago television, radio and print.

Months earlier, I had been reading a lot of books on advertising, marketing and how to become famous. I wanted to become a writer and an artist, and it seemed to me that fame for myself was a necessity.

I wanted to genuinely connect myself to a good cause. I was also depressed. Four young people I knew, friends, passed away. Three of them died of AIDS, and the fourth died of an aneurism, but I also heard he had HIV. These people never made it to the development of more stable and effective HIV drugs. I wondered how to connect my art with my activism.

Between 1995 and 1996, I had also been active in the Filipino community. I wrote an arts column for free for a monthly Filipino community magazine in Chicago. Soon enough I was also helping out to make the paper.

That era was just the beginning of digital or desktop publishing. We used both the computer and the traditional wax machine and paste-ups to layout the pages. I saw the fax machine roll out press releases every once in a while.

I saw politicians come to Filipino community social functions to campaign and win. I saw one politician come to the weekend parties that my publisher and I went to. I saw him win the first political position he was after. I saw people clap for him and vote for him. He is currently in jail for corruption.

I experienced the media and learned not to fear it.

One night, at about 3 am, I suddenly stood up off the bed, and had an epiphany. I had been reading a book by George Lois, the famous advertising expert who designed the iconic Esquire covers in the '60s and '70s.

One of his tips was that if two familiar symbols or concepts are joined together, a new but still familiar concept would result. This was how to get into the psyche of the public.

An idea came to me.

I had just recently read that the origami paper crane, which originated in Asia, had a belief or legend attached to it. It is said that if you make a thousand paper cranes, your wish will come true.

If I attached the red AIDS ribbon to the beak of the crane, it would symbolize many things. East meets West. AIDS Awareness. A wish for a cure. If white paper were used, it contrasted with the red of the ribbon. It looked like the dove with the olive branch. Hope. My idea! My creation!

Within a week, I issued a press release. Someone else from my community paper got ahold of my press release and she connected me with her nonprofit organization which had a budget for HIV/AIDS awareness.

My idea snowballed a little. I got two television interviews, one on the radio and a few local articles and mentions in print. I collaborated with two nonprofit groups.

I missed one radio interview because I overslept, and an appearance in a school because I got sick. I hate to say this, I lost the school contact's information. I pretty much did not show up.

I did a demonstration at a public library and another at a fashion show for AIDS Awareness. After about a month's worth of media attention, I was the one who backed out. I was not ready. It was a little too much for me, but that period was my baptism of fire in more ways than one.

I got my own domain and started making my website. By late 1998, when I moved downtown, I was able to post my AIDS awareness projects, ideas and articles. I posted pictures of the origami crane with the AIDS ribbon. I called it "The AIDS Crane."

About a year later, I got two important emails. One was from Australia and another was from South Africa. They were both from nurses. They both said they saw my idea online.

They both worked at their quarantined children's HIV/AIDS wards of their respective hospitals. Both of them got their young patients to fold the cranes and attach the AIDS ribbons to them. They strung and suspended the works like mobiles all over their units.

The nurses thanked me for the idea.

In my imagination, more stronger now than in the past, I consider them my children. My inspiration to continue caring and hoping. They fire me up and keep me going, even now.

That was the late '90s. I don't think those children are still alive. One can only hope and pray.

Dollman the Musical, A Memoir of an Artist as a Dollmaker, which I finished on Thanksgiving Day in 2011, and finished formatting on January 1, 2012 was written with sick and healthy kids in mind.

On special days when people were celebrating with their families, I preferred to be productive with my art and writing. It had always been this way.

And for these kids, when all is said and done, for all the kids of the world, I am The Dollman.

☙

I had this other idea too, way back. Picture this for yourself. My art priced at $1 million dollars. Maybe a painting or a drawing. Oh, what about my porcelain doll art?

My next art priced at $2 million dollars. The next at $4 million dollars. The next one at $8 million dollars.

This is me matching my art, math, business and economics. The rational here is that everyone gets to declare an increase in the value of their assets based on the last price paid. Even the second to the last buyer would be able to tell investors that the asset bought from me had at least doubled in price!

Way back in the past, I had thought about paintings and drawings. I kept my idea to myself, because I did not think paintings and drawings were competitive enough.

I had to justify why people would believe in me. There had to be more elements in the equation.

Then I thought about writing books from the perspective of an artist. Memoirs!

I wonder if four memoirs and my contemporary art dolls are enough. I have written four memoirs so far.

Here is my current version of this idea: I make 100 dolls with good backdrops and stands. With gold, rubies and diamonds.

The first 10 will be priced at $100,000. The next 10 will be priced at $200,000. The next 10 will be priced at $400,000. Then $800,000, $1,600,000, $3.200,000, $6,400,000, $12,800,000, $25,600,000 and the 91st to the 100th will be priced at $51,200,000.

If investors and investment companies respect the pricing, the price keeps doubling, the financial reports can say that the current value of their asset is at $51,200,000. This means that even the ones bought at $25,600,000 has at least doubled in value. The companies can sell the works to real collectors if they want to monetize the asset. While my work might take time, the paperwork can be immediately traded. With just a hundred art dolls, I would have contributed $5.12 billion dollars into the economy, circulating among the financial institutions.

I wonder if this idea could have saved the lives of those who committed "suicide."

It's a matter of just one investment company getting bit by this speculation... or I could be wrong, but if I succeed, I would have the U.S. and the Philippines being proud of me. If I fall flat on my face, the U.S. and the Philippines will not want to associate with me.

Whatever happens, it might become another memoir.

❧

It is 2014. I'm okay now. I miss my dad. I cry a little once in a while. I edit parts of this book and I tear up. I'm back to caring, despite the fact that I only have a hundred bucks on my person. I want to help the investment bankers. I imagine, what if I'm able to convince investment bankers to buy my art, with a geometric pricing schedule, will they be able to save their companies? I imagine that through my art, their financial statements return to be in the black. No more suicides.

Providence again. It is the 20th of February 2014. Mama and Dinna called as I was writing this chapter. It was daytime in Manila. February 21. They said they would send me pocket money for my birthday. I am turning 49 on February 23. I can stop worrying a little and continue to care.

Maybe you'll send me money. I'll make you a magical doll. It will change your life. And your financial statements.

Chapter 49

Counting Our Blessings

When I helped feed the poor on Thanksgiving Day, I was calm.

Papa died without suffering. I was told that he was never in pain. According to the doctors, pancreatic cancer visibly deteriorates a person and extreme pain is a major complaint.

When we caught up with each other in December, Dinna said Papa looked as if he was just sleeping. One of her requests to God was to preserve Papa's handsome face, and she believed she succeeded.

She was alone with Papa in the morgue when a huge entourage of people, from the parents to the siblings and children, to the driver and other relations, whoever else was there, townspeople, came down to the morgue with their dead.

They wondered why my sister was alone with Papa, no one was there to grieve with her. They compared their dead with hers. Theirs was deteriorated, ravaged by the disease and treatments.

They talked to my sister. They also said their relative had cancer, and they were surprised as to why Papa looked like he was just asleep.

Dinna told me that Papa had a "general confession" a couple of months prior. A general confession is when a person confesses to the Catholic priest his entire life's problems, conflicts and sins. Papa also had the last rites, the Sacrament of the Anointing of the Sick, but that is a given for Catholics.

Papa believed in miracles himself. He believed in what I did for him miles away, around the globe.

When I was in high school, he was a member of the Knights

of Columbus. He actually took me once and I was initiated into the group. I wasn't ready to keep coming back, but I had been initiated. I might come back in the future.

In 2006, when I attended Book Expo America, the annual convention for the publishing industry, I saw members of the Knights of Columbus picketing the movie, *The Da Vinci Code* on the sidewalk outside a movie theater. That year, the convention was held in Washington, D.C. While I found nothing wrong with the movie, I was elated when I saw the group, in their formal regalia that had a red cape, picketing.

Papa had also attended a *Curcillo* ("koor-SEE-yoh"), which is a 3-day sort of retreat training laymen to become Catholic Christian leaders.

Like I said earlier, in the late '80s, Tito Nick, Papa's younger brother, had an unknown illness. He was a doctor himself. He was either the dean or the chairman of a school of medicine in Manila. Papa and *Tito* Nick ("Uncle Nick") went to the same church of my grade school. He went to pray to the Virgin Mary, before the Lady of Lourdes statue, the same statue I faced telling the Virgin Mary about the bullying that was happening to me in school more than a decade ago.

He told me that as he prayed, he experienced a sort of vibration in his hand. He placed his hand on Tito Nick. Tito Nick's mysterious illness disappeared. Hospital tests proved it.

My request to God was complete and total healing for Papa. I would still say I succeeded, because I may had been instrumental with the pain issue, and I believed that whatever God allowed was okay by me.

Of course all this is subjective. No claims can be proven. In the end, we had our faith, not fact.

Comparing Papa's hospitalizations with what other Filipinos went through a month before, with thousands of people dying from Typhoon Haiyyan and the Bohol island earthquake, I was thankful.

My brother told me that I really cannot compare Papa with the other Filipinos. We should concern ourselves with our own family's well-being. Now that Papa is gone, we should even be more wary about our own kin. I agreed with him, but I have a habit of concerning myself with the plights of others.

By February, I no longer felt desperation. I didn't feel the need to go to church and hear mass every chance I got. I felt like it's over. Papa went to heaven. I finally was able to use my sewing machine and made fur coats for my doll art. I went back to writing on my laptop, and he I am finalizing my memoir about my art, Papa, healing and the strange.

I had come to appreciate my siblings more now. We were going to have to learn to watch out for each other and Mama.

In December, my brother insisted to treat me to the latest Nexus 7 tablet. He told me that I had been sending him a lot of stuff through the years, and he had never sent me anything in return. We went back and forth on the gift. I told him I did not need it, but he was insistent. He wanted me to have it before Christmas. It was important to him that I get it before the 25th.

We finally figured out how to get one to me. He sent me some money through Western Union. The Nexus 7 2013 edition on sale was nearby, at Microcenter. I had to reserve it online, and pick it up and pay for it at the store. On December 24, I picked it up. Photofinished gift! Thanks, Kuya Jing!

I can safely say that I had now gotten addicted to playing Candy Crush Saga on the Nexus tablet, just like millions of others all over the world. Not my brother. He said he didn't use his tablet for games. He uses it for presentations for his growing multi-level marketing business.

As I write this, it is the eve of my own birthday. Tomorrow is my birthday, February 23. I should celebrate. My brother texted me earlier today to greet me Happy Birthday and to tell me that he also just met his sales quota for his business, which entitled him to a free trip to Macau together with other top sellers.

CHAPTER 50

APOCALYPSE & ARMAGEDDON

Relax! Have a Seat! It's the end of the world!

My class in senior year high school had a religious retreat. I went to a Catholic school from prep, which was the grade before first grade, to high school. The university I went to, The University of the Philippines, was a state university, I'm just adding this, in case you're wondering. I did not have any classes in religion nor theology in college. Everything stopped in high school.

Back to high school. Senior year. My entire class of about 48 students went somewhere else for the weeklong retreat, still in Manila, to a facility run by nuns. I believe it was a week-long retreat. I think it was from Monday to Friday. I'm not sure anymore. There were talks and activities. Our chairs were placed by the walls of the room, a circular seating arrangement, so we all faced each other. We discussed religion and character education.

Each bedroom had two beds, so there were two people to a room. Ray was my roommate. My brother was our classmate, too, but he was in another room. In school, my brother and I had mutual friends we hung out with and Ray was one of them.

I want to tell you what I remember the most about the retreat.

☙

Everyday, in the morning, we had mass, officiated by a priest, of course. Every morning, the mass was not only for us visiting students. It was also mostly for the people in the area. I don't think the retreat house with that chapel took charge of a full-sized parish.

The people from the local area were supposedly poor. Most of them supposedly lived in the nearby squatters area.

I never saw them as that. They obviously showered and dressed nicely for the daily morning mass. That was dedication. They really did show up for mass everyday. Forget the way they dressed. They *showed up* for mass everyday.

However, here is why I'm writing about them now. The mass was in English, but the priest's sermon was in Filipino, so that the parishioners understood. The priest was white. He may have been European. Way back, that was something else to see.

I was one of the funnier people in the class. I knew a funny situation when I saw one. Some of us knew when to look at me to see a stupid reaction.

So this was what happened everyday. The white priest who spoke Filipino had a European accent, and so the way he pronounced Filipino words were a little bit rounded. His mouth sounded like it was hollow, like Audrey Hepburn with marbles in her mouth saying "The rain in Spain stays mainly in the plain" in the movie, *My Fair Lady*. Top that with the fact that he was a little rotund and, okay, here it is: he was cross-eyed.

And the people sang.

The seating arrangement in the chapel was traditional, using pews, which were where the locals sat. Being visitors, we had to add individual chairs in front of the pews in horseshoe fashion. So there were 48 chairs total distributed in front and on the two sides of the altar.

I was somehow placed right in front of the priest, so close that sometimes, his saliva sprayed on my arms.

And the people sang. There was a lady who led the songs. She used her right hand to conduct the rest of the flock so that they sang in unison. She sang clearly and loudly into the microphone. She was tone deaf!

As the priest spoke right in front of me, with his eyes crossed, his spit splattered me, I also noticed my classmates to his left and right sides, all laughing and looking at me, controlling my laughter, as my eyes watered.

Then the lead singer sang while moving her right hand in the 4/4 timing in music, as if she were the conductor, which she was, but she was out of timing and tone deaf.

What was funny about our class was that we were the smartest class of our year level. We took it upon a lot of us to join an interscholastic choral competition. We had one tone deaf classmate who joined our glee club. He was okay to join the singing group, for that last year in high school's last memorable bonding. He was told to keep it down.

From that first early morning mass, and the other morning masses, every morning, a good number of my classmates looked at me trying to contain my laughter. Everyday, I reminded myself that this was the territory of the good, respectable churchgoers who will be there for the years to come. None of the parishioners were laughing. They were seriously into the mass.

&

Flash forward to 2013. I had gotten older by more than 30 years. My dad was dying and I desperately prayed. I was in Chicago, where scandals involving priests had become so popular that some Halloween costumes can be dead on, satirical, totally disrespectful and sacrilegious, and very funny.

When I decided to go to daily mass in October, I got into counting how many people went. I sometimes counted 35. Only on Saturday mornings was I able to count past 40. I think those other churchgoers equated the short 30-minute Saturday morning mass with the hour-long Saturday afternoon "anticipated mass," which is equivalent to the Sunday masses. If they did, they were wrong. The Saturday morning mass is still part of the short daily masses. The obligatory mass was the one in the afternoon.

An anticipated mass is the next day's mass, which is said in the assumption that some people would not be able to hear the mass for that following day. Being that the Sunday mass is important, people like nurses, firemen and policemen who work on Sunday may hear the Sunday mass on Saturday. Most holy days of obligation will have an anticipated mass the day before.

Then winter came. This winter was bad. Since I was going to church more often than normal, I went to the Saturday morning, afternoon and Sunday masses. Once, as early as Friday, it was announced that there will be no mass on Monday morning because of the abnormally low temperature. I can't tell you how seriously devastating that was for me. True enough, the forecast for that Monday was accurate. I dared to walk outside. I came down with the flu.

I got familiar with the priests who said the daily masses. They all took turns to do it. There were three priests, the parish priest and two others.

There I was more serious than ever, asking for healing for Papa's cancer-stricken mortal body, and praying for the salvation of his immortal soul, and the daily masses, except on Thursdays, did not have pianists or organists unless the deacon was there. The parish priest, the deacon, the school choir and the school's music instructor were in tune.

The two other priests who said the weekday masses were not in tune. One of them was quite old, past 70. He was known not to take any salary from the parish.

I was just happy and thankful to our God, that we were all there, as few as 15 at times when winter came, and that included one or two nuns who lived in the compound and some laypeople who worked in the office.

The mass to me had become a celebration of so few people, that our singing, out of tune, untrained voices were to me, as precious, as magical and as heavenly as I would ever want us to have.

೧೦

I did my best to be inside the church between 7:15 a.m. to 7:30 a.m. so I can say the prayers from my prayer books and prayer cards. About two weeks before Papa passed away, I started to do the Stations of the Cross in church. I had been doing the

Stations of the Cross at home, but I tended to fall asleep.

The Stations of the Cross is a series of 14 images or carvings depicting 14 successive scenes from when Jesus was condemned by Pontius Pilate, to events as he carried the cross, to his crucifixion and death, to the 14th station, his burial. I wanted to get used to it, because the prayer can be tedious if your heart was not into it.

You have to go before each picture or carving, 7 on the left side of the church and 7 on the right, and each station has its own unique prayer, followed by one Our Father, one Hail Mary and one Glory Be.

This 14 Stations of the Cross now has a new, revised version. Pope John Paul II proposed to have a more accurate 14 Stations of the Cross. It will be a while before all the churches of the world replace the old.

There were three old Asian ladies who did the Stations of the Cross around November before the daily masses. They sat together during mass but they did the Stations separately before the mass. They stopped doing it by December. There must had been a common reason.

At the start, I prayed the Stations of the Cross at home. I lay on my bed and did it. I usually dozed off and continued where I left off when I woke up.

To do the Stations of the Cross "correctly," you not only should traverse the church, you also genuflect before each and every Station, as you say a short passage.

The Asian ladies, their version of supplication, was to actually kneel and then sit on the floor with legs parallel to each other, and bow so low that their faces almost touched their knees.

By late November, I started doing the Stations of the Cross in church. I did not want to get in the way of the ladies, so I did my best to beat them to it. I headed straight to the First Station as soon as I threw my scarf, gloves and beanie to the pew nearest the first station. I glanced to check their favorite pew to see if they had already arrived or not.

I made sure to be a few stations ahead of them. I'd pray fast if I had to. I sometimes overheard one or two ladies subvocalizing a few times. It was a little distracting. When you subvocalize, the letter "s" loudly stands out. Speedreading school forbids subvocalizing because it slowed down reading speed.

I did genuflect, but I felt self-conscious about it so this was one motivation to come much earlier. Better to be seen by only two to five parishioners than forty-five. Every time I genuflected, I positioned myself by the huge marble columns so that I was hidden from most of the churchgoers. Only when I got to the 12th to the 14th Station did I stop caring. By then, pretty much everyone who wanted to be in church were there. No thanks to winter, there were some days when I counted as little as 12 churchgoers.

Most of us were old and retired. The younger ones, myself included, were unemployed. There was one young guy who probably stayed in a homeless shelter. I could be wrong, but when we lined up for Holy Communion, with me behind him, he sometimes smelled of alcohol.

Well, the Asian ladies stopped doing the Stations of the Cross in December. I continued. One started to do it again this March.

Now they're all doing it again. I should be in church earlier again.

෴

One day I got out of my apartment, as usual, and walked to church. I knew it snowed the night before, and the forecast for the day was a little more dusting of snow and a lot of wind. I got to church early, chose a seat near the First Station of the Cross, took off my scarf, gloves and my beanie, a hat I knitted using a loom, and proceeded to the first Station to pray.

There was this really short, old, old, old lady who walked slowly and used a walker who went to daily mass. She came in later than I did. I was by the 10th Station, when this old lady passed by me. She was stooped and as tall as Yoda. She was so slow in walking, and as she moved, dragging that aluminum walker, she moaned continuously. And she farted as she walked, much like those squeaky shoes babies and kids enjoyed wearing. With intermittent farts, she heralded her arrival from the cold, coming towards me and passing by me. She passed gas all the way past myself and the other Stations I was going to pass by! I am supposed to genuflect, successfully reaching that optimal level of where the fart would be lingering, being that she was just a few inches taller than a ruler. And remember that church air does not move.

Now that ticked me off. In my mind I was saying she was an instrument of the devil. It was worse than if someone rode a bike inside the church while pressing a loud bike horn. When you become religious, you become sensitive to evil. The devil sends you signals and messages that he is not happy. I sensed evil.

Sure enough I did pass by the rest of the Stations. Did I have a choice? What if I suffered the wrath of God for not finishing the prayer because someone who walked so slow went ahead of me, assigning sacrilegious farts at each Station?

After mass, I headed out. It was very windy. It was a weekday, so there were cars on the street. About 200 feet from the church door, I passed by the same short, old, old, old lady. She was using her walker, and she was stopped.

As I passed by her side, she turned to me and uttered something I didn't understand. I thought she was Vietnamese. As she moaned out her possibly Asian words, probably assuming I was Vietnamese, she pointed to the semi-covered bus stop diagonally across the street. I understood. I asked if she wanted help to cross the street.

She nodded.

I got confused for a moment, wondering how to help her, because she pointed to the two-inch snow on the ground that stopped her light aluminum walker dead in its wheeled tracks. What was I to do? Her predicament reminded me of Tim Conway's character, "The Old Man," in *The Carol Burnett Show*. I was a bit amused and knew I was going to mention her in my book.

I looked at the street. It was rush hour on a weekday morning. There were cars, vans and trucks. The street had gotten busier than when I entered the church earlier at 7:15 a.m. It was the rush hour at 8:40 a.m.

I told her in a loud voice, pointing perpendicularly across that I will help her cross the street, directly across, and then, pointing to the bus stop, I told her I'll walk with her to the bus stop on the sidewalk. So my plan was to directly cross the street first.

I lifted the walker 2 inches from the ground. I felt resistance, as if the lady felt threatened that she would topple. We managed to get her walking. We crossed the street. I was smiling at the cars, on the left first as I and the lady crossed. The cars slowed down and stopped, and then the cars going the opposite direction slowed down as well. I kept smiling nicely, knowing obviously that they were all watching us do this death-defying feat, of crossing the snowy, slushy busy street on a windy weekday morning rush hour. How saintly of the old lady, going to church when she really should have just stayed home!

I don't know how old people think during rush hour, but she steered her walker diagonally towards the bus stop! Her intention was to make everyone wait even longer! I was so embarrassed. I was not self-conscious like when I genuflect in church, I just felt like this lady, who was stooped and as tall as Yoda and as slow as The Old Man, got her way and bullied me to help her block the flow traffic, possibly causing the course of history and the economy to change via her butterfly effect, by diagonally traversing the road for about 120 feet. Granted that she probably figured out that the sidewalk might have all that loose snow as well, and the road had been driven on, with the snow flattened. I was just glad no one blew their horn at us. We probably stopped 20 cars on each side.

When it was over, I, Superman, the great superhero who just got finished with the good deed, decided to pass by Jewel, the grocery, to get a couple of freshly baked, cheaper, grocery-priced donuts before I went home!

The next day, I went to church again. I sat on my pew after my usual Stations of the Cross. Mass was to start in 5 minutes. One of the Asian ladies who used to do the Stations turned around to look at me. I smiled and nodded my head. She stood up and walked towards me.

"Thank you for yesterday!" she said.

"What do you mean?" I asked back.

"I saw you helping the old lady cross the street. I want to tell you that the two of you looked like a beautiful picture together, with you helping the old lady cross the street to the bus stop," she said.

"Oh that was nothing," I replied. She smiled and walked back to her seat.

∽

This isn't really the end of my story. I am leading this to my view. I listen to this radio program, Coast to Coast AM and other related paranormal programs. I had been listening to talk about ghosts, UFOs, conspiracies, doomsday scenarios, prophecy, the coming of the Messiah, the apocalypse, Armageddon.

I was getting familiar with the other churchgoers. We looked like a ragtag group of characters in a Stephen King movie, where we, as main characters were supposed to save the world. If we had visions of the apocalypse and Armageddon, I'm sure we would all be called by the unknown force, good or bad, to find a way to show up in some cornfield that had a small shack where an unfamiliar old lady was waiting.

∽

What I'm asking is, "Where is everybody else?"

How come no one but 15 to 35 people attend daily mass? How come there have been more empty spaces than parishioners on Sundays? A lot of pews are empty!

I made this comment to a few friends. One person even asked me why would I even begin to go to church? She talked about priest scandals, and so I should not even go to church!

Well, when I decided to reconnect with God, Papa was sick. I came to the conclusion that I cannot let my relationship with people get in the way of my relationship with God.

I had improved. Despite my funny look at us churchgoers, I now find each churchgoer precious. Every single day I was at church was a triumph. When I sang the church songs, I whisper and eat my words sometimes. I let others carry the tune, even if they were tone deaf. I thank God for their presence.

I no longer felt the need to be in church everyday. Maybe Papa and the others I had started to pray for, had gone to heaven. Maybe I can become less and less consistent in going to daily and Sunday mass.

I'm still funny.

☙

The advent of spring, March 2014. The weather had gotten better. The parishioners are back. Attendance to the weekday mass has increased.

I haven't seen the short, old lady in a while. She went to church when not too many did. I pray for her now. I hope she's okay.

Chapter 51

Convenience & Last Resort

When I called my cable company to complain about their prices for my internet connection, they instead offered me a deal where for the same price, I can have cable tv. I said okay. How great thou art! I was so easily convinced.

I didn't care for television anymore, so it took me three weeks to connect the cable box they sent me. I opted to do it myself.

Mama had always told me all she watched was EWTN, the Catholic network. I checked it out.

That day, the station featured a live telecast rally in Washington, D.C. They were against abortion. I guess that puts a date on this chapter, Wednesday, January 22, 2014, the 41st anniversary of Roe vs. Wade, the landmark Supreme Court case that legalized abortion in the U.S.

A few women had the courage to come up to the interviewer, telling the viewers that they opted to keep their babies and offer them up for adoption, because life was precious. When asked who was the father, at least one of them said it was a one-night stand.

If I were critical, I would have had the opinion that the lady should not have had sex in the first place.

What if I was a parent and that was my daughter. How would I feel?

I tell people I'm gay, and I write about being gay as well, then I also say I'd also fallen in love with women, I can even name them, but my point is, to some people, simply being gay is evil.

I can't say I'm a rah-rah activist. I would not go to rallies. I would rather stay at home and write about my own views. Writing books have a permanence to it. Rallies and demonstrations are important as well. I go to church not just to connect with God by receiving Holy Communion, but to connect with other people. I felt that it was important to worship with other people.

It's difficult to choose sides with issues. I have my own views but I don't really want people to side with me.

I have my own twisted parables.

☙

Once upon a time, someone came up to a preacher.

"Hi Preacher how you?"

"Oh, I'm just fine."

"How's your daughter?"

"Oh, she's just fine."

"Is she still living with you?"

"No, she's living elsewhere."

"Oh she's living alone."

"No she's with her other half."

"She's married?"

"No, she's cohabiting with her boyfriend without the sanctity of marriage. She's a lucky girl. The man is a doctor."

"How is your son?"

"Oh, my son's going to hell. He's gay. I threw him out of my house! If God can throw people out to where there's gnashing of teeth forever, then so can I."

"Oh no!"

"Shall we go in? I think it's time to go to the Pick and Choose Church and worship the God of Convenience. Service will begin soon, and I can't wait to give my sermon."

☙

"Hey whatsup?"

"I have a headache."

"Where are you heading?"

"I'm going to the drugstore to buy some pain medication."

A week later:

"Hey whatsup?"

"I have a stomach ache."

"Where are you heading?"

"I'm going to the drugstore to buy some stomach ache medication."

A week later:

"Hey whatsup?"

"I have cancer. It's terminal."

"Where are you going?"

"I'm going to church to ask for a miracle."

"Oh I'm going there too. The one two blocks away and to the right."

"Yeah, the Church of Last Resort."

☙

I have gay friends and acquaintances who view sex as just another exciting activity. When we talked about it, we talked as if we were normal about it.

I'm no saint neither. I reconnected with God because Papa had cancer. I started praying for relatives and friends, some of whom had been dead for decades, only after I decided that I should probably pray for them since I was already praying for my dad.

Just because I had been going to church lately does not mean I'm newly totally against anything I used to do. This supposed memoir, with weird and more religious stories and introspections does not make me cleaner and holier than anyone, nor does it make me so much better than myself in the past.

I should had asked the psychic surgeon to elaborate some

more on his sexual practices, that despite his beliefs and daily life, he still was able to do what he was able to do.

I knew he told me he did not worship the Virgin Mary.

My understanding about the Virgin Mary, is that as Catholics, we did not worship Jesus Christ's mother. We pray to the Virgin, in just the same way as we pray and talk to our dead relatives while in prayer. We ask the Virgin to help get results from God.

It's the same as when someone goes to a protestant pastor who does not worship the Virgin Mary and asks for prayer.

☙

"Hey Pastor!"

"Hey whatsup?"

"My wife is sick and dying."

"Oh, don't worry. I'll pray to God so she would get better."

"Thanks Pastor! I really would appreciate that. I had thought about asking the Virgin Mary to pray for my wife as well."

"Oh no, we don't do that. You can't ask her to pray for the health of your wife. She has no power to do that. She's just the mother of God."

"But you do? You will pray to God for a miracle for my wife?"

"Of course! I will pray for your wife's health. And that's a promise."

☙

My bachelor's degree in Biology taught me a simple lesson: that we are biological, physical beings, and if we hurt ourselves, we will feel pain. If we infect ourselves, we will get sick. If the infection comes from having sex, then so be it.

Basically, it does not matter if we are straight or gay, it's what we do that is the issue. If we keep pursuing sex, we can get sick from it.

People are like Lemmings, the game. They move about where they are allowed to be in. If gay people are discouraged from settling down, then they don't have that option. Because that avenue is blocked, they will go elsewhere and do something else.

※

That friend of mine who passed away of HIV/AIDS whom I volunteered to lay my hands on. He got the disease from being promiscuous. He loved what he did. He kept doing it. He got sick, after which he became a speaker in HIV/AIDS awareness panels. He started to consider himself an activist, truthfully telling people what he did to get the disease, among others.

I was conflicted with visualizing to make him better. I had no assurance that he will change his ways. He had no assurance that psychic healing worked.

The problem with psychic healing, is that it is unprovable for the most part, and to change what seems to be fun, because of a belief system based on faith and conjectures is a question of which comes first, the chicken or the egg?

Should we change first and then ask God for healing, or should God heal us first before we change?

Should we ask proof that He exists to become more faithful?

※

I discovered that in the prayer books, the word "mercy" is abundant. My interpretation related to mercy was that, as we live our daily lives, we may be unknowingly doing things, thinking thoughts and taking stands that God never approved of. That's probably one reason why we should keep asking Him for mercy.

I personally keep asking God for mercy just in case, because even now, I don't know what he wants from me, nor do I know for a fact that he did anything for me when I was asking for Papa's cure. I just went ahead and set in my mind that God was powerful enough whether He decided to help me or not.

Sometimes, I thought of a funny joke and I laugh. Maybe God heard it and thought it was funny too. Nevertheless, I still remind myself that God can be wrathful. I should also fear Him.

Some people think that doing good deeds won't get you to heaven. Simply by believing that Jesus is the Saviour and believing that Jesus had already saved them is the way to heaven. Some vehemently believe this.

The above belief makes sense, but it reminds me of this next twisted "parable."

☙

"Hey Madonna's coming to town to do a concert."

"Oh nice, thanks for telling me."

"I'm going to get a ticket and see the show. I wanna be there, watch and hear the music, and rock it out with the crowd! Wanna come with me?"

"No. Just knowing Madonna is coming makes me feel like I am already there."

☙

One of the churches gave away a book, *Rediscover Catholicism* by Matthew Kelly. He wrote that despite the scandals by wayward clergy, we should remind ourselves that it was the Catholic clergy who introduced to the general public healthcare, education and adoption among other important things that we now take for granted.

☙

The psychic surgeon also had this idea: What is stopping us from writing the Third Testament? There's the Old Testament, then the New Testament, but why should the story stop there?

He told me that if I went to the bookstore, for example, with all the technology and knowledge we had accumulated, do not all the books represent a Third Testament?

I agreed with him then, and I still agree with him now. If the Bible stopped with the New Testament, then doesn't that make us okay just to become followers, as opposed to being followers AND leaders?

The psychic surgeon and I talked close to 30 years ago. This possibility of a Third Testament, being in the back of my mind, had, through the years, been one of my earliest and strongest motivation to write about my views and my life.

It's not that I thought I was special. It's that I think everyone should do it.

☙

In the Bible, Jesus was asked what he thought about the eye for an eye passage? In reply, He said that there is a new rule. If a person strikes you on one cheek, turn the other cheek.

Well, Christ left 2000 years ago, and now we follow the rules of our denominations. Some concepts changed again.

☙

I heard of a story, where this priest, who had been canonized a saint after his death, made an announcement, while he was still alive, to his people, that those who attended a certain church event would get some sort of grace.

As the people were partying, he suddenly had a revelation. God told him that only two of the attendees would get the grace.

The priest realized that he made a mistake. How can he tell that to the people?

What if we were wrong in our assumptions?

☙

Maybe we should continually pray, ask for God's mercy, to forgive us in case we happened to be making a mistake in the way we think we should live our lives and worship and follow Him?

What if the Gates of Heaven will only open up for us once, and only once?

Are we taking a chance feeling safe with our own convenient interpretations?

What if we got certain things wrong?

☙

Dear God of Convenience and Last Resort, Thank you for letting us pick and choose what is right and wrong for us and for those we prejudge before your final judgment.

The end.

Chapter 52

Riddles

In an earlier chapter, a teacher of mine mentioned Cain's question to God, "Am I my brother's keeper?"

That to me was a riddle, personally for me. My answer is, right now, unequivocally: YES, but it took me years to realize it.

In 2008, my sister and I had a really bad argument that I literally threw her out of my place. We'd forgiven each other since. I cannot believe what got over me to become that selfish, knowing full well that she was not from Chicago. At the same time, she never told me what her own inner conflicts were. It took her six years to let me know what really happened.

Our aunt became mean to her from the moment she went in with her luggage. Our aunt had passed on. When Aunt Li came home to the Philippines to die, she and Dinna had the chance to be okay again. Dinna opted not to tell me anything, and so did my aunt. It's a long story, but now it's over.

In 2011, I let someone stay with me, and then I threw him out as well, but the circumstances were different. So here I go again, with the "but." There always seems to be a justification of that moment where we draw the line so that we will continue looking like we were still righteous.

Lately I had expanded my range. If I wanted to "ascend" enough to become a healer, I started playing with this thought: Who is my brother? Who would I tolerate as my brother?

I thought, if I were Abel, and Cain whacked me in the head, and there I was, a ghost floating in the air. If I had learned my lesson right, it would be that I should forgive Cain for killing me. He may have made a mistake, but I still would not want him to go to hell. I should forgive him for his misdeed.

I have expanded my thought exercise a little more now. Maybe I should train my mind to see that all the rest of the world is my brother. Will I let just about anyone whack me in the head?

※

I had not yet told you that I also pray for the angels. I'm confirming this now, before I end the book, just in case you want to become a healer. I wanted to become a healer and I prayed to and for the angels.

The Bible mentions angels, and the Catholics recognize the hierarchy of angels, classifying them into nine groups. Whenever I walked to church, I pray one Our Father, one Hail Mary and one Glory Be for the daily purposes of the angels, naming each group, so I would have said the three prayers nine times by the time I entered the church two blocks away.

So there would be the seraphims, cherubims, thrones, dominions, powers, virtues, principalities, archangels and guardian angels.

Supposedly, the thrones look like flying wheels. Some ufologists say that they could be ancient UFOs, misinterpreted to be angels. I am into UFOs and the paranormal. I still pray for the thrones. I may be praying for the safety of the UFOs. I'm okay with that. I'll just keep praying.

The last group are the guardian angels, and supposedly, all of us have been assigned at least one, including people we don't like. Only lately was I able to think that I was also praying for the angels of my enemies and other people I didn't like. So here was my limit in my mental exercise:

I have yet to get used to the thought that I was also praying for the angels of my enemies and people who disliked me.

Lately, I made the declaration that I was praying for the guardian angels in existence of all beings in the universe and other dimensions, not just humans on earth. When I did that, I stopped thinking about my enemies.

༼༽

Like what was mentioned in the Bible, it's easier to talk to and care about strangers than your own friends and family. Even Jesus was condemned and crucified by his own people, but well-received all over the rest of the world. There's a riddle.

༼༽

I discovered I prayed better if I told God at the start of the prayer to forget about me, and that I was praying for everyone else. Sometimes I got the feeling that getting graces for myself was not how God wanted me to pray.

Sometimes I say, "If I get any good graces from this prayer, please give it to my dad or someone else who needs it more."

There's the double edged sword here.

What if, the more I say "Forget me, God, I'm praying for others," the more God will favor me?

Then again, what if I come to heaven's gate, and they say, "Well, you did not earn enough graces, because you requested for God to give all your graces away?"

༼༽

Here's another riddle. The Rapture compared to the Titanic.

In the movie, *Titanic*, some people stayed behind. They knew they were gonna die. To allow others in the lifeboats was a noble choice.

On the other hand, a lot of Christians think they will be raptured or saved simply because they had accepted Jesus as the Savior.

I have never heard a preacher nor a priest tell anyone to ask God to leave them behind in exchange for someone they love to be raptured.

Lately, the concept of the rapture seemed to me like the ultimate "Me first!"

Are we really going to heaven if we have a "Me first!" attitude?

Is it really heaven we are going to, if, as we get beamed up, we look back to see our loved ones being left behind?

☙

Some radio personalities talk about how bad propaganda is and that conspiracy is everywhere. They seem to be in the right.

Then they say they are concerned about the end times.

Then they talk about being religious, the Rapture and what people can do to go to heaven.

Then they mention homosexuality and that people are going to hell just for being gay.

That's propaganda right there, they are using it themselves, just like the people and groups that they are against.

They associated with issues that seemed to be good and righteous and for the good of the majority. Then they throw in something extra in the grocery bag.

That's a riddle.

☙

These are my own riddles.

If you want to become a psychic healer, based on the teachings of the Filipino psychic surgeon I encountered, you will encounter more and more riddles. Your own riddles. More questions than answers about how to become not just a psychic surgeon but a good person.

Faith is faith. It cannot become fact.

I did the best I can to become a healer for Papa.

I'm sure I made mistakes along the way.

Maybe I rushed it for him.

Maybe I did not do enough.

Maybe I succeeded. Maybe I did not.

What riddles will you have?

CHAPTER 53

WORDS

I'm not saying I'm a very good writer. I can claim that I have improved. I continually study how to write. I have also spent hundreds of hours studying hypnosis for two reasons: The major reason is that hypnotic principles can be incorporated into writing. The minor reason is that I felt the need to understand it as it is "possibly" used on the sick. I still believe that psychic surgery and psychic healing use hypnosis. Then again, even doctors use hypnosis as well.

As a writer, I know my weaknesses. Prepositions, idioms and tenses confuse me. This book is self-published. Amel is an editor. I once asked her to edit my work. She was good, but I felt that my voice disappeared in her own style of writing. English is my second language. I did my best.

*

As I end this book, I have to let you know that even now, I believe that psychic surgery, psychic healing and faith healing is a combination of faith, hypnosis, self-suggestion, autosuggestion, and the placebo effect. The skin opens up because the will and faith to do it is strong.

*

Catholics have what I call "formulaic prayers." Prayers that have already been written for our convenience. Recite and repeat.

My appreciation for words is reflected in my interest in published prayers. The prayers were written and worded in a way that would not have occurred to me. The words and the play of words are actually hypnotic. They trigger something in the psyche.

There were days when I decided to spend ten hours praying.

The only way I was able to do it was to recite or read those prayers in the prayer books and prayer cards. There was no way I could have spent ten hours ad-libbing and extrapolating on my own.

I would encourage you to look into reciting formulaic prayers.

An entire mass is formulaic. There is a reason for this.

☙

When I was praying for Papa, I reworded the prayers. I did not say, "Our Father who art in heaven, hallowed be Thy Name... Give us this day our daily bread and forgive us our trespasses, as we forgive those who trespass against us..."

I said, "Papa's Father, who art in heaven... Give Papa this day his daily bread and forgive him his trespasses, more than he has forgiven those who have trespassed against him..."

I reworded prayers as I thought might be helpful for him.

Maybe I'll get excommunicated for mutating, and adding my own DNA to the church prayers.

What it did was it made it more personal. I was saying my own prayers. It made me more alert. My heart was in it.

Find your own ways to make yourself alert. Find your own ways to get God to notice you. I would not know how to do this, really. What I had were interpretations.

Faith is faith. It will never fully become fact.

CHAPTER 54

HOW TO BECOME A PSYCHIC SURGEON

Before anything else, if you have any mental problems, or if you have been diagnosed with a mental problem, or even if you only think you have one, I would suggest not looking into becoming a healer until you are well. Just read all this like you are doing now. Don't attempt to proceed because it's not healthy and it will only worsen your condition.

Sometimes, we believe something to be true, too strongly, that we do not allow for the possibility that we might just be delusional and we do not realize we are already hurting someone else or ourselves.

There's a warning label.

You should also read on the "Messiah complex." Wikipedia defines it as follows:

"A messiah complex (also known as the Christ complex or savior complex) is a state of mind in which an individual holds a belief that they are, or are destined to become, a savior."

I cannot say I have the messiah complex. I might have the Jonah and the Whale superduper procrastination complex. I implied that I procrastinated so long to get a book on psychic surgery written, which is true, that even though I procrastinated, it got written anyway.

The problem with me, is that I studied writing and art, and I made sure that I can deliver both. I think the messiah complex has something to do with delusions, again, without supporting tangible proof.

At the same time, I'm still doubting myself. Maybe what I have produced in terms of art and writing are not good enough yet to make me collectible.

☙

I'm ending this memoir of an artist as a healer with this chapter, because chances are you bought this book because of your curiosity of how it is to become a psychic surgeon, or you really want to become one. I had gotten *my* way, you've read the memoir of an artist as a healer. The least I can do is to give you a few more pointers to patch up loose holes.

Return to my definition of faith healing, psychic healing and psychic surgery. Psychic surgery will only manifest itself after a period of time when you can confidently say you *are* a psychic healer. However, to become a psychic healer, you need to connect with the Higher Power who just happens to be God, and that means that you need to have faith. There's a fine print for you.

We are also under the assumption that I, as the author, actually witnessed psychic surgery, which I did. This is what has given me confidence in writing all this. I'm reminding you once again, that the premise that genuine psychic surgery exists, is a given.

Do not plan to go to the Philippines looking for a guru who will teach you the ropes. Try this book first. Not all Filipinos are good. Some can trick you, some can kidnap you. If you venture into the forest, you'll get bit by a snake before you see a bigfoot, an extraterrestrial being or a UFO, or their Filipino counterparts.

This is important: All this is about faith. I am 99.99% sure that it will remain so. I have no desire to prove anything. My goal was to write a memoir and it's done. If you like to experiment, maybe you have a grant, then see what you can prove. I hope you find answers and discoveries.

Remember Padre Pio, the saint who had stigmata and was also seen to have levitated and bilocated? He manifested these things without the need to approach anything scientifically.

My next suggestion for you is to read the Lessons from a Psychic Surgeon chapters all over again. Then read my other chapters and analyze how I interpreted his lessons. I said I "failed" because

I was not able to heal my dad 100%. However, he had pancreatic cancer and never felt intense pain until he died. Use my efforts as a way to calibrate yours because you may have to do more than what I did. Or try something I had not tried.

You must also take note that I did not do everything that the psychic surgeon told me to do. I may have missed something.

Yes, I did miss something. I did not read the Bible. I thought Papa's condition needed prayers and a miracle, more than devoting time for my own period of enlightenment. I should have started to read the Bible years ago.

Go back to work, or do whatever it is you do to make some money, make preparations, and then have your own interpretation of 40 days and 40 nights of being with God and everyone else in His camp. Or maybe concentrate on God and Jesus Christ alone.

If you think you can pray at night and then go back to normal in the morning, then do so, and see how much progress you can make. If that's what you can do for now, I'm sure God or that higher power, will understand that that is your starting point. When I discovered that anyone can bring home and store holy water, I did so. I have two bottles at home.

Here's a strange thought: If God urgently needs a lot of soldiers for some upcoming battle, you might be surprised at what you can do.

Make a list of what you think you should do to become "miraculous," however you define that word to be. I bought prayer books, attended mass, wore the scapular, wore a blessed cross, attached some tiny religious medals, also blessed, to the cross, etc. I did not mention I wore a cross, but I do wear a blessed cross.

I clutched a crucifix and a rosary when I slept as if they were teddy bears. It was comfortable for me when I did it and I felt like I was on a mission. I also felt like doing it as much as I could. The rosary was a gift from Papa and I visualized connecting with him through it.

I had stopped doing it now that Papa had passed on. Well, I

would not mind doing it, but right now I had been busy with my art and writing. My muse had come back. God probably wants me to finish this book. Lately, I had been rushing to sleep and waking up in a hurry to get back to my laptop.

Read on the lives of saints and see what they did, and see if you can do what they did.

List the good and bad things that you do in your life. Imagine placing them on adjustment bars with knobs and sliders on them, like mixers in a recording studio, that you can move left and right. How do you think you should adjust those?

Expect strange things to happen. Some invisible forces will not like what you are up to. Don't communicate with invisible beings. There's a reason we cannot see them. I never did that and I don't encourage you to do that either.

Miracles happen, but it obviously takes time. Do not be impatient. It can take years. Even Christ waited years before he was able to perform miracles on a regular basis.

Learn to keep this a secret. Treat the invisible like a spouse. Treat God like the ultimate spouse. He won't incriminate you if you won't incriminate Him.

Don't claim to be a healer. The FDA will come after you. Claim to be a psychic healer or a faith healer. Claim to be a religious person. Tell people you can do laying on of hands and you can pray for healing for the sick person.

Actually, before the FDA can even stop you, your own denomination or local church, family and friends might be the first one to stop you. You might be perceived as misrepresenting your church. I could be misrepresenting the Catholic church.

This is why you should not declare what it is you do. Even your church, which is based on faith, will dispute all this, which is also based on faith. This is why you need to learn to keep this a secret.

Learn to shut up. Sometimes neighbors would prefer to have "normal," average people around them.

Tell people that if they are taking prescription medication, they should keep taking them, because faith healing is an unsubstantiated activity based on belief.

Your faith should be enough even at the beginning.

Do NOT ask a sick person, "Do you believe in God? Because I will heal you through the power of God, but only if you believe He will heal you." You are putting the person on the spot and making him or her desperate to say yes.

Don't use someone's desperation to your advantage.

Learn to sense negativity and negative energy and avoid them. If you are reading this and you are new to this, suffice it to say that you are not ready to be visible, lead and change the world and that you might not be able to defend yourself from the negative.

You might notice some people's attitudes towards you change in a negative manner. Become aware and avoid them.

Learn to avoid psychic vampires. They can drain your energy. Learn to say no to them in a nice way.

Do not become confrontational.

Some bad souls can sense a good soul.

Leave friends and family members alone unless the situation is desperate. They won't be pleased with your "faith experiment." They will think you are weird.

Learn to say no. "No, no, no!" You are not here to please people.

A sick person is not an opportunity to do wonders. There will come a time when you feel compelled to "help," but the person or people did not ask for it. What will you do in such a situation? It's your call.

If you really want to do this, learn to not drain your physical, spiritual, mental and emotional energy by having sex. Learn how many days you can do without it. Sorry.

You will notice that some of the things you do, or like to do, or some things you do to other human beings, and others, and certain ways you think, however you interpret all this, might need to be curbed.

Do not charge. If people want to give you something, that would be good. If they are rich, and they give you little, that's insulting. They want their cake and eat it too.

You need to come to agreements within yourself and with others that feel honest and caring in your gut. Otherwise, your psychic healing energy will not flow anyway. It will all be a waste of time, and you would know in your gut that the best thing to do is walk away.

Some people can easily be swayed. Do not mislead people.

In the future, maybe we can form an organization. We cannot form a cult. I want to remain Catholic. You might want to remain something else. I think that would be good.

See first if you can stop headaches, migraines and other types of pain. I would stick to that for a while.

Remember that some treatments might need repetition.

If you are into satanic worship or something related, and you know that strange things have happened, try "switching sides" as an experiment. It could be fun. God, angels and other good beings exist, too, I think.

Don't attempt psychic surgery. Don't use sharp objects. Don't use your spit. Don't use candles and other fire hazards. Don't hold snakes. Don't attempt exorcisms. Don't preach unless you're already a minister or priest. Make sure your hands are clean. Use alcohol. Wear clean surgical gloves. Always wash your hands after touching another person.

Don't claim to be the Messiah, some people will believe and follow you.

∽

Thanks for reading my book!

LET'S CONNECT ONLINE

Email
valzubiri@gmail.com

Facebook Fan Page
http://www.facebook.com/pages/Val-Zubiri/137514462978637

Facebook Page
http://www.facebook.com/val.zubiri

Twitter
http://www.twitter.com/valzubiri

Blog
http://vzubiridollman.blogspot.com

LinkedIn
I use vzubiri334@aol.com for LinkedIn
please use this email when the form asks you
for my email address

Phone
Available upon request by email

www.ingramcontent.com/pod-product-compliance
Lightning Source LLC
Chambersburg PA
CBHW020853180526
45163CB00007B/2490